Transforming Healthcare

Healing You, Me, and
Our Broken Disease-Care System

Transforming Healthcare

Healing You, Me, and Our Broken Disease-Care System

Kim Evans, APRN

Butler Books
Louisville

ISBN: 978-1-941953-75-4
Printed in the United States of America

Book design by Carly Schnur

Published by Butler Books
P.O. Box 7311
Louisville, Kentucky 40257
phone: (502) 897-9393
fax: (502) 897-9797
www.butlerbooks.com

To all healthcare providers who are committed to transforming our healthcare system to a model based on wellness and disease prevention, delivered with love and compassion.

To each of you who have believed in our vision of wellness and in creating your own optimal health of mind, body, and spirit.

Contents

Introduction | ix

CHAPTER 1: The Emperor's New Clothes 1

CHAPTER 2: Creating Healing Environments
for Patients and Families 23

CHAPTER 3: Creating Systems that Support
All Providers and Caregivers 35

CHAPTER 4: Being Your Own Patient Advocate 51

CHAPTER 5: Integrative Medicine:
A New Paradigm for Practice. 73

CHAPTER 6: Shifting to True Healthcare:
Preventive Integrative Medicine. 87

CHAPTER 7: Self-Care: Modeling and
Creating Healthy Behaviors 107

CHAPTER 8: A New Paradigm for Elder Care 141

CHAPTER 9: How Do We Make Healthcare Affordable? . . 155

CHAPTER 10: Transforming Healthcare: Healing You, Me, and Our Broken Disease-Care System 173

Acknowledgements | 195

Bibliography | 197

About the Author| 211

Introduction

Have you visited your doctor or primary care provider recently? Was your wait time to see your provider longer than the actual office visit? Did you feel that more attention was given to the computer in the room than you as the patient? Was more time and energy spent on collecting your insurance information and determining how you were going to pay for your appointment instead of focusing on the nature of your office visit? Did you have a higher out-of-pocket expense for your visit than previously, despite paying much more money annually for your "health" insurance?

Are you disillusioned with "healthcare" in our country right now? Do you feel like you are paying more for healthcare but receiving less? Is your primary care provider happy with the system in which she or he works? Does your provider seem stressed and overwhelmed with all the changes in healthcare? What is happening to our healthcare system?

Let's take a look. The term "healthcare" is actually a misnomer. The truth is we really do not have a healthcare system. We have a disease-care system. Healthcare professionals wait until you get sick with a disease and then try to fix your disease. This is despite the fact that seven out of the top ten diseases that kill Americans are chronic illnesses, of which more than half could be prevented.

Do you feel healthy and well? Do you know that you could be healthier if you made some different decisions or changed some unhealthy patterns in your life? Are you aware that true health and wellness is beyond just physical health? True wellness means not only having healthy bodies, but also healthy minds, emotions, and spirits.

Have you or your family member been hospitalized recently? Did you feel like a family member needed to stay with you or your loved one to help if hospital staff were not available? Did you find it beneficial to have someone there with you or your loved one to ensure no errors were made in the care provided? Were you or your family member able to receive quality sleep? Was the food healthy and nutritious? Were adequate care or instructions provided when you or your family member left the hospital?

The focus for our healthcare system has shifted and many institutions have lost sight of their primary goal, which is to help people become healthy and treat those with illnesses or traumatic accidents. Instead, the focus is predominantly on the almighty dollar, the bottom line, and who is going to pay the bill. While the importance of money cannot be ignored, it should not be the primary focus for healthcare institutions.

Not only are patients and families disgruntled about our current healthcare system, so are providers. Many providers are leaving healthcare altogether. Some providers, in an effort to contain their costs, have sold their practices to hospitals or healthcare system. These mergers have not always resulted in happy marriages.

Our healthcare system is broken in many ways. My intention in writing this book is to share a vision of transforming healthcare: healing you, me, and our broken disease-care system by:

- Redirecting the primary focus of health to wellness and disease prevention

- Creating models of health that prioritize patient and family needs above all else

- Creating healthy team-based systems that empower and inspire all providers as valued members of the team, recognizing each one's expertise and contribution for the patient, from physicians to housekeepers

- Providing guidelines so you can achieve your own optimal wellness of mind, body, and spirit

- Demonstrating a sustainable payer system that will meet healthcare expenses for individuals and families without bankrupting anyone, including our country

Sooner or later, each of us will interact with the healthcare system and providers, whether for our families or ourselves. Let's create a system that we can be proud of, and that we would feel confident and comfortable in taking our loved ones to for health and healing. Let's transform healthcare into a system of true healing, caring, compassion, and wellness for all.

CHAPTER 1

The Emperor's New Clothes

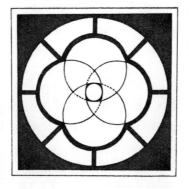

Our healthcare system is in trouble. We spend more money per capita than any other industrialized nation in the world. This might be tolerable if our outcomes were the best in the world. Sadly, our outcomes are not near the best—especially with chronic illnesses and infant/maternal mortality in childbirth.

Regarding Healthcare in the United States

- The United States ranks 37th out of the 40 top nations for best health system according to the World Health Organization report on health systems, 2000.[1]

- America was rated 29th in infant mortality (behind Cuba) by the Centers for Disease Control and Prevention.[2]

- The United States ranks last among the top 11 nations for healthcare efficiency, equity, and outcomes despite spending more on healthcare than any other country.[3]

Why is our healthcare system so broken? Here are the key contributors that I believe lead to a dysfunctional healthcare system:

- Overemphasis on the "bottom line"

- Prioritizing provider needs over patient needs

- Primary focus on physical issues only without inclusion of psychological, emotional, and spiritual aspects of health

- Autocratic, physician-centric structure of healthcare institutions

- Overemphasis on pharmaceutical and surgical approaches to treatment

- Fear-based legalistic culture

- Disease-care models with little priority on prevention, wellness, and wholeness

- Current trends in today's healthcare

Let's take a brief look at each one.

Overemphasis on the Bottom Line

Many hospital administrators don't want to see the truth. They believe that as long as the bottom line is strong, and the hospital is making money, everything is fine. It's as if they are as oblivious as the townspeople in the fable, "The Emperor's New Clothes." While focus on the bottom line cannot and should not be ignored, neither should it be the predominant focus. Hospitals are intended to be places of healing and recovery, not profit centers benefitting from the ill health of the populace.

Several years ago, while working as a critical care clinical nurse specialist, I encountered a patient in the intensive care unit who was very ill and who eventually died. She was a close relative of a hospital administrator across town. Two days before the patient died, one of our hospital administrators came to visit her family. He wanted to offer a "courtesy discharge," which meant the patient or family did not have to stop at the cashier's office to pay the bill before leaving the hospital. My first thought, knowing the gravity of the situation, was that the only discharge the patient would receive would be a celestial discharge. This saddened me that the administrator's idea of comfort was a monetary gesture. This was one of my first epiphanies that the hospital's focus was misdirected.

On another occasion, the hospital would not allocate funds to have emergency crash carts placed on each floor (the carts hold essential items to use when a patient's heart arrests or they stop breathing). However, they did allocate funds to purchase a cherry wood table for the administrative conference room and to remodel the administrative area to build two separate bathrooms so six to eight men and women would not have to share one. Another local hospital, in order to meet their budget, eliminated 80 ancillary help positions. Within the same week, the hospital purchased brand-new office furniture for their newly hired director of risk management, despite the fact that new furniture had been purchased just three months earlier for the previous director of risk management. When asked about these disparities, administrators responded that funds were allocated from separate budgets. This confused me since all departments are part of one institution. Again, these actions seemed to be out of alignment with the overall hospital mission and miss the mark of the hospital's true purpose: patient care.

Prioritizing Provider Needs over Patient Needs

When I worked in the hospital, I observed that laboratory blood tests were drawn between four thirty and six thirty in the morning. This continues to be common practice today. A bright light disrupts the patient's sleep as the phlebotomist collects the blood for ordered tests. It was done early in the morning so that the results were back on the patient's chart by the time the physician or nurse practitioner made rounds. This practice was originally done to ensure that these providers could do hospital rounds early and then make it back to their offices to see patients. Today, most hospitals now employ hospitalists (doctors and nurse practitioners who are trained to care for patients while they are hospitalized) and therefore do not have to leave to go to an office. However, the practice of obtaining blood work or X-rays at very early hours and disrupting a patient's sleep continues. Obviously, this is not a system that prioritizes the patients' needs; otherwise labs and X-rays would be conducted at more normal waking times.

I also observed how most therapies were conducted between eight in the morning and four in the afternoon. During these hours, some patients had three to five therapeutic treatments such as physical therapy, occupational therapy, or speech therapy. After four thirty, there were no further therapies until the next day. Ideally, patients should have a therapy session and then be allowed to rest adequately before their next treatment. Healing could be expedited if therapies were more evenly spaced throughout the entire day and evening, with adequate rest periods between therapies. Again, the hospital systems' priorities were placed above the patients' needs.

In my position as a critical care clinical nurse specialist, I commonly found a large gap between clinical research and practice. For instance, the nursing and medical literature has supported open visitation for families of patients in the critical care units since the early 1980s. Most patients are comforted and more relaxed when family members are present. Even though large numbers of studies continue to support open visitation, there are intensive care units across the country that still restrict visitation times for families. Why do these units resist changing practices when evidence clearly supports the benefit of open visitation?

I observed that some nurses seemed to feel threatened by having family members present in the intensive care unit while they were caring for patients. Other nurses felt that spending time answering families' questions took time away from the patient. I found that educating nurses about the research results and the benefits for patients of open visitation usually helped allay the nurses' fears and resistance. Training nurses in communication skills also proved beneficial.

A common response that I received when I would question practices that were out of alignment with current clinical research was, "Well, we've always done it that way." In most cases, it appeared that people were simply resistant to changing the current practice. Effort, time, and resources are necessary for hospitals to bridge the gap between clinical research and practice. This must be prioritized to ensure that patients receive the best care supported by current evidenced-based research.

Primary Focus on Physical Issues Only without Inclusion of Psychological, Emotional, and Spiritual Aspects of Health

Most of Western medicine is built on a reductionist model, Koch's postulates, in which we break things into smaller and smaller parts to determine a root cause. Without a doubt, this model has served us well in many ways and led to many life-saving discoveries such as:

- The cause of many infections

- Effective antibiotics against some of these infections

- Multiple pharmaceutical compounds for varying diseases

- Technological advances such as the creation of coronary stents or balloon angioplasty for blocked coronary arteries

- Multiple advances in surgical and anesthesia techniques

However, as our knowledge in both science and medicine has progressed, it has become obvious that the reductionist model has limitations. Larry Dossey, MD, has described the evolution of medicine and science brilliantly as progressing through three eras.[4]

The first, Era I Medicine, describes health and illness as completely physical in nature. The focus is on finding the right combination of drugs, technology, and medical treatments to cure the patient.

Era II Medicine acknowledges the mind-body connection and the growing awareness that a person's consciousness (thoughts, emotions, and beliefs) has an impact on one's physical well-being.

Era III Medicine describes the latest evolution and has developed out of scientific discoveries in quantum physics, which have proven the non-local nature of consciousness. Our minds and spirits are not limited to our body (or brain) and are described by Dr. Dossey as non-local.

Our minds, thoughts, and awareness are unbounded and infinite in time and space. We can no longer view the body as a machine powered by the mind. Humans are complex, integrated, infinite, dynamic systems and so the attempt to break things down to smaller and smaller parts to find a single root cause (reductionist model) is not only impossible, but irrelevant. Quantum physics has negated our whole way of thinking.[5] Previous research methods of double-blind, placebo-controlled designs have been beneficial in identifying single causes or effects of an intervention. However, modern research methods will be better served if there is a focus on exploratory designs and outcomes-based inquiries that can acknowledge humans as integrated, dynamic systems.

Clearly, we are more than just the "sum of our parts." Not only do physical, psychological, emotional, and spiritual aspects affect our health, but also do family, social, community, and environmental aspects. Still, the focus of conventional medicine remains predominantly on physical issues.

Over and over, I witnessed this in my role as a critical care clinical nurse specialist. When we began open-heart surgery in our hospital in 1996, a pilot trial project of art therapy was incorporated. An art therapist saw every patient who had a myocardial infarction (heart attack) or coronary artery bypass surgery (open heart surgery). The results were astounding. Seventy-five percent of these patients had significant unresolved grief issues. These patients literally had experienced a "broken heart," and then physically, they experienced a blockage in their coronary arteries. In one case, an elderly gentleman had suffered a heart attack complicated by congestive heart failure.

He was discharged, only to be readmitted two to three times over the course of eight weeks. Further investigation revealed that this man had recently lost his wife of 60 years. While his physical care had been met, no one had addressed his grief or his psychological or emotional needs. These unmet psychological and emotional needs clearly exacerbated his physical issues. I knew we were missing the mark by only focusing on patients' physical aspects without addressing their psychological, emotional, and spiritual components as well. For a person to truly heal, all components of well-being must be recognized, acknowledged, and addressed.

Autocratic Physician-Centric Structure of Healthcare Institutions

Hospitals are not considered safe places. In 1999, the Institute of Medicine (IOM) sent a "wake-up call" challenging all hospitals to improve their safety standards when they published a report documenting that up to 98,000 people die annually from medical mistakes.[6] A more recent article cited that medical errors now account for the third leading cause of death and claim 251,000 lives each year.[7] The numbers of those injured are even higher, which is estimated at forty times more than the death rate.[8] Why is this? Why does every major organization not only allow, but also recommend that patients have someone with them while they are hospitalized?

Certainly, hospitals have made progress since the initial IOM report in 1999, with safety initiatives, procedure manuals, case management, and evidence-based practice standards. However, the progress has been slow to change systems. The reason is that many hospitals are still governed in autocratic, authoritarian, physician-centric models, which sometimes cater to the needs of physicians and practitioners over the best interests of patients and other providers.[9] Systems based on these models can lead to fragmented

8

care, poor communication, lack of consistency in provider practices, and lack of standardization of protocols or procedures based on evidenced-based practices.

Traditional biomedical models may devalue other providers by creating a hierarchical structure with an imbalance of power of physicians over other providers. This model can leave other providers feeling powerless, frustrated, and oppressed. For instance, in traditional biomedical models of care, other disciplines are not even included in the care of the patient until an order is written by the physician eliciting their services even though each of these disciplines has their own body of science and knowledge. When other provider services are requested, these disciplines commonly operate in "silos" with little communication among the practitioners, which can lead to fragmented care.

The reality is that systems are not going to change until radical shifts occur in institutional cultures toward patient-centric models— models in which each discipline contributes its unique expertise and is valued as an important part of the healthcare team. In patient-centric models, members of the healthcare team interact in non-hierarchical relationships working together for the patient's best outcome.

Why are hospitals so slow to change? The culture of "We've always done it this way" is very prevalent. It's similar to a fish in the ocean that becomes so accustomed to the environment that it doesn't even see the water. We have become so used to dysfunctional environments in healthcare that we believe it's the norm. As healthcare providers, we are all guilty of being the "Emperor," oblivious that there is even a problem with the culture, let alone addressing the need to change the culture. Let's explore the impact of an autocratic authoritarian system on the largest group employed within the healthcare system—nurses.

The nursing profession is a classic example of an oppressed group. Common characteristics of oppressed groups are feelings of powerlessness that might include frustration, negativity, cynicism, and depression. Oppressed groups resort to behaviors of horizontal violence, stabbing each other in the back or "eating their young." Any seasoned nurse has witnessed any or all of these characteristics exhibited at one time or another by other nurses. These behaviors escalate the dysfunction, frustration, and burnout in healthcare settings. I have witnessed new nurses treated so poorly by seasoned nurses that the new nurses leave the nursing profession altogether, downtrodden and defeated. We must change this.

Most of my nursing colleagues have great ideas on how to change the system and the culture. They are ready to embrace patient-centric models and bring healing compassionate care back into the healthcare system. Yet there are barriers. One of my colleagues, a great nurse, had the gift of making each person, whether patient or family, feel heard and supported. Sadly, not only was her gift unrecognized by her nurse manager, but the nurse was in fact, reprimanded by her supervisor for "taking too much time" with her patients. We must create a culture in which compassion is not only supported, but also is welcomed, valued, and becomes an integral part of the institution's function. We are not going to change healthcare until we change the present culture and shift to a patient-centric model, where every member of the team is equal and valued for their unique contribution to the patient's care and well-being.

Overemphasis on Pharmaceutical and Surgical Approaches to Treatment

There is no doubt that pharmaceuticals have contributed greatly to our modern healthcare system. The advent of penicillin, cephalosporins, and other antibiotics, has helped eradicate many infectious diseases. Vaccinations have completely obliterated some diseases that used to plague us (pun intended), such as tuberculosis, smallpox, diphtheria, and polio. Yet, have we gone overboard on pharmaceuticals and vaccinations usage? Today 88 percent of people older than 60 are on at least one prescription medication, and 37 percent take five or more prescriptions.[10] This presents a safety issue. The more prescription medications one takes, the greater the likelihood for side effects to occur.

Other startling statistics involving children and adolescents document that more than 22 percent of children under 12, and 30 percent of adolescents are on prescription medications.[11] Thirty years ago, prescription drugs were rarely used for adolescents. Most clinical studies on pharmaceuticals only include the adult population and do not address safety and efficacy for pediatric populations. Yet they are prescribed for children and adolescents anyway.

Why do we rely so heavily on pharmaceuticals? Some believe it's related to the massive marketing done by pharmaceutical companies. Marketing expenditures for pharmaceuticals in the United States have increased by 20 percent every year since 1997.[12] Our medical culture has conditioned patients so that when patients seek medical attention, they expect to get a prescription and may even feel slighted if none is given. Over 75 percent of provider office visits and close to 80 percent of outpatient and emergency room visits involve some type of prescription drug therapy.[13]

The United States is the only country that exhibits this heavy reliance on prescription drugs. Most other countries first use other types of treatments such as herbs, homeopathics, teas, and essential oils. In my practice at the Institute for Integrative Medicine, we use many herbal and homeopathic formulas that are effective, less expensive, and have fewer side effects than pharmaceuticals. In America, there still exists a significant bias against nutraceuticals and natural formulas. For example, many of us are familiar with the recent warnings against using bisphosphonates for osteoporosis due to an increased incidence of jaw necrosis.

Integrative Therapeutics, Inc. has two supplements, Osteoprime and Ostivone that work synergistically to reverse bone loss caused by osteoporosis. These formulas are safe, well tolerated, and lack the significant side effects of bisphosphonates. Despite clinical studies (including some conducted 19 to 24 years ago) to support their efficacy, most women are offered only bisphosphonate options from Western medicine practitioners.[14] Is this bias influenced by the control, domination, and marketing of pharmaceutical companies? I think that's a great possibility.

Surgical procedures have also become a mainstay in Western medicine and in many cases, are lifesaving. However, there are potential risks with any surgery. Sometimes there may be less invasive options that should be attempted before jumping into surgery. For instance, it is well documented that chiropractic care is a great treatment for spinal disc subluxations.[15] Surgical interventions for disc problems such as a laminectomy or spinal fusion may be avoided if effective chiropractic care is utilized.

Fear-Based Legalistic Culture

Many healthcare recommendations use fear as a tactic to coerce patient compliance. For example: You better eat healthy or you'll get heart disease and have a heart attack. You must have a colonoscopy to ensure you don't have colon cancer. If you are female, you must have a mammogram to ensure you don't have breast cancer. If you are male, you must have a prostate-specific antigen (PSA) test to make sure you don't have prostate cancer.

I am not implying that screening tests are unimportant; however, the implications and reasons for these tests are all fear-based—to make sure you don't have the big "C"—cancer. Yet we know that cancer doesn't just happen all of a sudden. Many inflammatory and immune processes happen long before a tumor or cancer cell develops. What if we focused on healthiness and how to support and improve our immune systems in addition to the screening tests?

Let's go back to breast health. Mammograms are actually late indicators of breast cancer. Thermal imaging scans, on the other hand, reveal changes in breast health eight to ten years before these changes will become apparent on a mammogram.[16] Also, evidence exists that for some women, there is greater risk when having a mammogram due to radiation exposure than the benefit of identifying breast cancer.[17] Since thermal imaging requires no radiation exposure, it is very safe. In my own case, I had a thermal imaging scan done in 2005 that showed inflammatory signs in my left breast. I eliminated processed foods, high fructose corn syrup, and hydrogenated oils from my diet. I began to eat a predominantly plant-based diet with fish and occasional organic chicken. I also made the following changes to enhance my breast health:

- Eliminated caffeine since I have fibrocystic breasts

- Used a deodorant without aluminum

- Avoided bras with underwire

- Did a dry brushing technique to improve lymphatic flow

- Did self-breast massage to improve circulation and lymphatic flow of the breasts. My colleague Betty Greaver quotes Cheryl Chapman when she refers to this as "phluffing the girls."[18]

Since I made the above changes, I have had eight repeat scans, all of which have been normal.

Did my interventions prevent a possible occurrence of breast cancer? This answer is unknown. I do know that my breast health has improved without an exposure to radiation. Why is thermography not widely used and recommended in Western medicine? When I researched the reasons, I found significant undertones of political and economic implications.[19] Not surprisingly, organizations such as the American Cancer Society, whose funding depends on promoting mammograms, do not recommend thermography. An increased use of thermal imaging studies might decrease income generated by radiology departments. Despite ample research documenting the positive benefits of thermal imaging, including the fact that it is non-contact and pain-free, involves no radiation exposure, and is comparatively portable, the recommendation of thermography for breast cancer screening has been limited in the United States.[20]

Politically there has been an effective influence to keep mammography as the gold standard despite evidence that mammography is a late indicator for breast issues and that repeated exposure to radiation from mammography might actually be a causative factor in breast cancer incidence.[21] There is also an underlying (in this case, I believe exaggerated) fear among Western medicine practitioners to recommend anything outside of traditional medicine for fear of being sued if something goes awry.

I was reminded of the fear-based legalistic culture that is so prevalent in healthcare when I had a recent surgical procedure. I had developed some abnormal tissue on my labia and my OB/GYN nurse practitioner suggested laser therapy to eradicate the abnormal growths. The surgical consent form included the following: "I understand that some aspects of the surgical procedure or significant surgical tasks (harvesting grafts, dissecting tissue, removing tissue, implanting devices, altering tissue, wound closure, etc.) may be performed by an assistant(s) other than the primary surgeon/practitioner physician identified in on [*sic*] this consent. I further understand and consent to one or more of the assistants (assisting surgeon, surgical assistants, and other healthcare providers, residents/students, etc.) who may assist or perform one or more of the significant surgical tasks referenced above."

It goes on to read:

RISKS OF PROPOSED OPERATION/PROCEDURE

My physician has explained the reasons and benefits of the surgery/procedure, significant alternatives, the risks involved, and the possibility of complications to me, and my questions have been answered. No guarantee or assurance has been given as to the results that may be obtained from this procedure.

1. I understand that any surgery/procedure involves some risks. The more common risks include infection, bleeding, nerve injury, blood clots, heart attack, allergic reactions, severe blood loss, risks of blood transfusions (discussed in #10), and other risks described by my physician. These risks can be serious and possibly fatal.

Keep in mind that I was having a simple laser procedure involving no incisions. I quickly realized that the hospital used a generic surgical consent form, to cover any and all procedures and operations, and all possible negative outcomes, most of which were irrelevant for me. Despite knowing that this consent form was a catch-all, and having an extensive background in healthcare, I felt scared to read that consent form moments before going into the operating room.

I started crossing out all the parts that were irrelevant to me such as harvesting grafts, dissecting tissue, and implanting devices. It wasn't until later that I realized that by signing the consent form, I had also given permission for "one or more of the assistants (assisting surgeon, surgical assistants, and other healthcare providers, residents/students, etc.) who may assist or perform one or more of the significant surgical tasks referenced above." This means that I could have had a surgical intern, resident, or student do this procedure with my consent. I was so anxious when reading the consent form that I didn't even realize at the time what I consented to. And I am familiar with consent forms.

The pre-op nurse was patient with me. Usually patients are given these consent forms and are not expected to read them in their entirety. Patients are shown where to sign and initial their consent. If one takes time to read the form to learn what they are signing (as any prudent person should), they are often treated with disgust, impatience, or intimidation because they are taking too much time to sign the consent form and prolonging the pre-operative phase. I know the pre-op nurse was grateful when she could administer the sedative that would relax me before the surgery. When she brought it, I asked her if she thought I needed the entire amount. She said, "Honey, if anyone needs this, you do!" It's too bad that the healthcare culture is so fear-based and legalistic. I would have been much more relaxed if the consent form had said, "Today you are having laser surgery. We will do everything we can to ensure a successful outcome and to make you comfortable during your procedure. In rare instances (less than 2 percent), things don't go as expected. Please know that we have a highly trained professional staff that will intervene immediately in those rare instances." Imagine a system with a culture of comfort, wellness, and healing instead of the predominant, fear-based, legalistic culture.

Disease Care Model with Little Priority on Prevention, Wellness, and Wholeness

It bears repeating that most Americans are acutely aware that we do not have a healthcare system. Instead we have a disease-care system. Healthcare professionals wait until you get sick and then try to help you. This is costly, both for our healthcare system and for our own health and well-being. Until the reimbursement policies change, and more money is allocated to disease prevention, health practices, and behaviors, we will continue to have a disease-care system that is ineffective and expensive. We have all heard the old adage, "An ounce of prevention is worth a pound of cure." This could not be more apropos than in healthcare. Here are some examples of why we must shift our system to health and wellness instead of disease care.

As a critical care specialist in 1995, one of my responsibilities was to run the pulmonary rehabilitation program. We had data to support that when patients with chronic obstructive pulmonary diseases (COPD) participated in a six-week pulmonary rehabilitation program, their admission rates to hospitals decreased annually over 60 percent. Medicare covered a hospitalization, which, at the time, averaged about $10,000, but Medicare would not cover the $650 for these patients to participate in the rehab program. Today, 21 years later, there is still underutilization and poor reimbursement for pulmonary rehabilitation programs despite these programs being recognized as evidenced-based care for COPD patients.[22]

Similar examples can be found with many other chronic illnesses. For instance, one of the worst complications for patients with diabetes is poor circulation in the extremities, which can lead to the need for a leg amputation. Medicare will cover the cost of the amputation but not the education for proper diabetes management to prevent the need for an amputation. In patients with heart disease, cardiac rehabilitation is only covered if a patient has had a myocardial infarction (heart attack) or coronary artery bypass graft surgery (open heart surgery). While these patients definitely need cardiac rehabilitation, wouldn't it also make sense to offer heart healthy education to those with a history of heart disease in their family? We know that proper nutrition and exercise can prevent, eliminate, and decrease inflammatory responses in the body that are associated with the three biggest killers of Americans—heart disease, stroke, and diabetes.

Thirty percent of all cancers can be prevented with proper nutrition and lifestyle measures.[23] Healthy nutrition and exercise are two of the most significant intervention strategies for disease prevention. Yet as Andrew Weil, MD, states, "Most healthcare providers are functionally illiterate when it comes to nutrition." This is because most medical school programs only include 30 minutes to three hours on nutrition. Usually the "nutrition education" simply includes when a patient should be referred to a registered dietician. We must change this. Most people expect to be able to get health information (especially nutrition) from their primary care providers. Yet, if their providers are not educated in nutrition, patients are at a loss for proper guidance. A recent article supports the need to reform medical school curriculum to include implementation of healthy lifestyles, of which nutrition is an essential component.[24]

Current Trends in Today's Healthcare

The primary objective for the Affordable Care Act of 2010 (ACA) was to provide coverage for most Americans to receive healthcare, given that 43 million had been uninsured or underinsured. Many hoped that the ACA would create change in our healthcare system, affording a much greater focus on wellness and disease prevention. Disappointingly, the system remains predominantly focused on disease care. Attention has only shifted toward asking who is paying for the care. The predominant, expensive, and ineffective disease-care models remain. Whether the threatened repeal or replacement of the act, with even more limited provisions will occur, is unknown at this writing.

Another potentially dangerous trend is the number of physicians and nurse practitioners who have sold their practices to hospitals. Once a provider's practice is owned by a hospital, the provider loses their autonomy and must adhere to the politics and policies of that institution.

One of my friends is a cardiologist. He sold his practice to a local hospital that made him an attractive offer, including benefits such as a retirement plan and health and long-term care insurance for him and his entire staff. After about a year, the hospital began to exert pressure on him to reach and maintain a certain quota for invasive coronary angiograms (heart catheterizations). This pressure has caused him undue stress and emotional upheaval. No longer are his care decisions strictly based on clinical indications. Now he must factor in meeting the hospital administrator's demands to perform a minimum number of procedures.

I foresee a dangerous trend here. What if a patient presents with potential coronary symptoms, and the cardiologist hasn't met his quota of heart catheterizations for the month? Might he lean toward doing the invasive procedure—even when it's not clearly indicated? Performing heart catheterizations when they are not completely indicated increases risks to patients and increases overall healthcare costs.

When another friend of mine sold his primary care practice to a local hospital, the administrators told him there would be no influence from the hospital on his medical practice. After several months, the hospital (which was owned by a Catholic institution) mandated that providers could no longer write prescriptions for birth control since this was in direct conflict with the Church's doctrine. In order to provide optimal patient care, the group that my friend was with ceased their contract with this hospital and joined a competing local hospital. My friend felt that his own values and ethics to provide optimal care for his patients were compromised by the hospital mandate, and he chose to affiliate with an institution more closely aligned with his own values. I applaud physicians and nurse practitioners who choose to maintain their own private practices despite the economic burdens and to maintain the integrity of their values and beliefs despite the challenges.

By now you can appreciate several factors that are contributing to our broken disease-care system. It's time to give up the illusion of the "Emperor's New Clothes," acknowledge the problems in our healthcare system, and face them head on. Let's imagine what it would look like if we transform these components of our current disease model into a healthcare system that is truly based on patients' healing, wellness, and disease prevention with care and compassion as the foundation.

---

1. World Health Organization, *The World Health Report 2000—Health Systems: Improving Performance* (Geneva, Switzerland: World Health Organization, 2000).

2. Andrew Weil, *Why Our Health Matters: A Vision of Medicine That Can Transform Our Future* (New York: Hudson Street Press, 2009).

3. Karen Davis et al., "Mirror, Mirror on the Wall: How the Performance of the US Health Care System Compares Internationally," *The Commonwealth Fund* (2014).

4. Barbara Montgomery Dossey and Lynn Keegan, "Nursing: Integral, Integrative, and Holistic: Local to Global," in *Holistic Nursing: A Handbook for Practice*, 6th ed., eds. Barbara Montgomery Dossey and Lynn Keegan (Burlington, NH: Jones & Bartlett, 2013).

5. Kimberly A. Evans (Genevieve Bartol and Nancy F. Courts, original authors), "The Psychophysiology of Body-Mind Healing," in *Core Curriculum for Holistic Nursing*, 2nd ed., eds. Mary Helming, Cynthia C. Barrere, Karen Avino, and Deborah Shields (Burlington, MA: Jones & Bartlett, 2014).

6. Linda T. Kohn, Janet M. Corrigan, and Molla S. Donaldson, "To Err Is Human: Building a Safer Health System," (Washington, DC: Institute of Medicine/National Academies Press, 2000).

7. Martin A. Makary and Michael Daniel, "Medical Error: The Third Leading Cause of Death in the US," *BMJ* 353 (May 2016): i2139.

8. Ibid.

9. John J. Nance and Kathleen M. Bartholomew, *Charting the Course: Launching Patient-Centric Healthcare* (Bozeman, MT: Second River Healthcare Press, 2012).

10. Nicholas Bakalar, "Prescription Drug Use Soared in Past Decade," *The New York Times*, October 18, 2010, https://www.nytimes.com/2010/10/19/health/research/19stats.html; and Qiuping Gu, Charles F. Dillon, and Vicki L. Burt, "Prescription Drug Use Continues to Increase: US Prescription Drug Data for 2007–2008," *NCHS Data Brief* 42 (September 2010): 1–8.

11. Gu, Dillon, and Burt, "Prescription Drug Use."

12. Nick J. Fox and Katie J. Ward, "Pharma in the Bedroom ... and the Kitchen ... The Pharmaceuticalisation of Daily Life," *Sociology of Health & Illness* 30, no. 6 (September 2008): 856–68.

13. National Center for Health Statistics, "Therapeutic Drug Use," Centers for Disease Control and Prevention, https://www.cdc.gov/nchs/fastats/drug-use-therapeutic.htm, accessed October 23, 2017.

14. Anne Schaafsma, P. J. F. de Vries, and W. H. M. Saris, "Delay of Natural Bone Loss by Higher Intakes of Specific Minerals and Vitamins," *Critical Reviews in Food Science and Nutrition* 41, no. 4 (May 2001): 225–49; Marjo H. J. Knapen et al., "Three-Year Low-Dose Menaquinone-7 Supplementation Helps Decrease Bone Loss in Healthy Postmenopausal Women," *Osteoporosis International* 24, no. 9 (September 2013): 2499–507; Domenico Maugeri et. al., "Ipriflavone Treatment of Senile Osteoporosis: Results of a Multicenter, Double-Blind Clinical Trial of Two Years," *Archives of Gerontology and Geriatrics* 19, no. 3 (November–December 1994): 253–63; Donato Agnusdei and L. Bufalino, "Efficacy of Ipriflavone in Established Osteoporosis and Long-Term Safety," *Calcified Tissue International* 61 (1997): 523–27; and Xin Zhang et al., "Effects of Ipriflavone on Postmenopausal Syndrome and Osteoporosis," *Gynecological Endocrinology* 26, no. 2 (2010).

15. Jonathan Murphy et al., "Improvement in a Patient with Disc Protrusion and Extruded Fragment Following Subluxation-Based Chiropractic Care: A Case Study and Selective Review of the Literature," *Annals of Vertebral Subluxation Research* (November 2015): 178–83; Michael Burcon and Jennifer Pero, "Resolution of Glossopharyngeal Neuralgia and Spastic Dystonia Following Chiropractic Care to Reduce Upper Cervical Vertebral Subluxation: A Case Study," *Journal of Upper Cervical Chiropractic Research* (January 2014): 7–13; Nathan Berner and Don Capoferri, "Complete Cervical Kyphosis Correction and Resolution of Low Back Pain Utilizing Pierce Technique," *Annals of Vertebral Subluxation Research* (November 2011): 183–88; and Christine M. Goetz, et al., "Adding Chiropractic Manipulative Therapy to Standard Medical Care for Patients with Acute Low Back Pain: Results of a Pragmatic Randomized Comparative Effectiveness Study," *Spine* 38, no. 8 (April 2013): 627–34.

16. Vinitah Sree, E. Y. K. Ng, Rajendra U. Acharya, and O. Faust, "Breast Imaging: A Survey," *World Journal of Clinical Oncology* 2, no. 4 (2011): 171–78; and Eddie Y. K. Ng, "A Review of Thermography as Promising Non-Invasive Detection Modality for Breast Tumor," *International Journal of Thermal Sciences* 48 (May 2009): 849–59.

17. G. J. Heyes, A. J. Mill, and Monty W. Charles, "Enhanced Biological Effectiveness of Low Energy X-rays and Implications for the UK Breast Screening Programme," *British Journal of Radiology* 79, no. 939 (March 2006): 195–200.

18. Cheryl Chapman, *The Happy Breast Book: A Women's Guide to Keeping Your Breasts Healthy and Happy* (Maplewood, NJ: Cheryl Chapman, 2003).

19. David Bowman, "What the Research Says about Thermography: An Annotated Bibliography of Research on Using Thermography for Detecting Breast Cancer," Thermal Imaging of the Southwest website, http://tiofsw.com/wp-content/uploads/2014/08/Scientific-Bibliography-Mammograms.pdf, accessed October 23, 2017.

20. Ng, "Review of Thermography"; Heyes, Mill, and Charles, "Enhanced Biological Effectiveness"; Bowman, "What Research Says about Thermography"; Muffazzal Rassiwala et al., "Evaluation of Digital Infra-Red Thermal Imaging as an Adjunctive Screening Method for Breast Carcinoma: A Pilot Study," *International Journal of Surgery* 12 (December 2014): 1439–43; and Nimmi Arora et al., "Effectiveness of a Noninvasive Digital Infrared Thermal Imaging System in the Detection of Breast Cancer," *American Journal of Surgery* 196, no. 4 (October 2008): 523–26.

21. Ng, "Review of Thermography"; Heyes, Mill, and Charles, "Enhanced Biological Effectiveness"; and Anouk Pijpe et al., "Exposure to Diagnostic Radiation and Risk of Breast Cancer among Carriers of BRCA1/2 Mutations: Retrospective Cohort Study (GENE-RAD-RISK)," *BMJ* 345 (2012): e5660.

22. Sam Birnbaum, "Pulmonary Rehabilitation: A Classic Tune with a New Beat, but Is Anyone Listening?" *Chest Journal* 139, no. 6 (2011): 1698.

23. Michael S. Donaldson, "Nutrition and Cancer: A Review of the Evidence for an Anti-Cancer Diet," *Nutrition Journal* 19 (October 2004).

24. Robert F. Kushner et al., "Nutrition Education in Medical School: A Time of Opportunity," *American Journal of Clinical Nutrition* 99, no. 5 (2014): 1167S–73S.

CHAPTER 2

Creating Healing Environments for Patients and Families

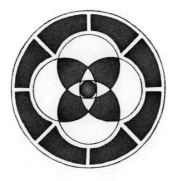

Patient-Centric, Healing-Oriented Hospitals

In 2003, I had the privilege of visiting the North Hawai'i Community Hospital in Waimea, on the Big Island of Hawai'i. This hospital is a model of what future healthcare institutions can be. The 50-bed hospital was built under the direction of Earl Bakken. He was the previous CEO of Medtronics, which is a company that manufactures pacemakers. He has always been a visionary with heart. Even as the

CEO of Medtronics, he knew the importance of connecting hearts beyond paced rhythms. Despite the highly technical aspects of the pacemaker industry, he found a way to include human connection and compassion. Annually, he would sponsor a dinner for his engineers who developed the pacemakers and the patients whose lives were transformed by the technological genius of these engineers. These were often tearful, emotion-filled encounters.

When Bakken retired, he moved to Waimea on the Big Island of Hawai'i. The community recognized his visionary talent and asked that he help them build a hospital in their community. At first, he resisted since he had just entered retirement. But being the visionary he is, the thought of building a new hospital intrigued him. He helped lead a phenomenal effort to realize the dream.

First, he brought together all the healthcare leaders in the area, including practitioners of Western medicine, traditional Hawaiian medicine and alternative medicine, physicians, acupuncturists, nurses, and kahunas (local traditional healers) to participate in the planning process. Together, they researched the area to find the best location energetically to build such a hospital. They chose an area with exquisitely beautiful scenery surrounded by five mountain ranges.

The hospital is built in a semicircle so that each patient's room has a sliding glass door that opens out to an herbal healing garden with the mountains in the background. The rooms are constructed so one enters the patient's room at the foot of the patient's bed, which is parallel to the outside wall. Patients can look out the sliding glass door and see the mountains or look at the wall at the foot of their bed adorned with beautiful scenic pictures. This design ensures that the patient is not facing the hallway and decreases the patient's distraction by preventing undue stimulation from hallway activity. Patients experience more rest and relaxation. The hallways are wider, and the ceilings of the rooms are higher than the standard eight feet found in most hospitals, thus reducing the fight-or-flight feeling common in most institutions. This design promotes calmness and relaxation for patients and visitors.

The lighting is full-spectrum instead of fluorescent. This natural soft lighting provides a calming effect. Beautiful artwork is displayed in every room, again helping to allay patient and visitor fears and foster a peaceful healing environment. All the treatment rooms contain paintings of beautiful scenes. The paintings are located with the patient in mind. For instance, in the radiology department that houses the CT scanner, a beautiful mural of clouds and a blue sky is painted on the ceiling. How thoughtful for the patient staring upward when the CT scan is performed.

I was most inspired by the head of the dietary department. She explained that she trains her kitchen staff to have awareness that they are not only cooking food for patients; they are also creating healing energy with food. She shared that if any of her staff feels upset, is frustrated, or has any negative feelings while preparing food, she insists that they leave the kitchen area to take a moment, breathe, and regroup before returning to food preparation. This way, the kitchen staff intentionally brings only positive healing energy into the meals they are making. This approach provides amazing results in both food quality and in the healing capacity of the food being served.

Each of the nursing staff at the North Hawai'i Community Hospital is trained in complementary modalities, such as music therapy, healing touch, aromatherapy, guided imagery, Reiki, and other energy-based therapies. The intensive care units and operating rooms have windows, so that patients and staff can maintain their day-night orientation, which is critical to maintaining the body's normal circadian rhythms. Much attention is focused on making patients, family, and staff comfortable.

The Planetree Network

North Hawai'i Community Hospital should be the model of how we can create healing environments in hospitals by placing patients' priorities foremost. Other hospitals on the mainland have instituted similar philosophies and designs for creating such environments. The Planetree Alliance is a nonprofit organization begun in San Francisco in 1978 that partners with healthcare organizations to help them create patient-centered systems and healing environments.[1] Hospitals within the network, for instance, have focused on how to create healing environments in the décor and design of their hospitals. Décor is certainly an important aspect of creating healing environments, but Planetree recognizes that what is most important is the caring, compassionate atmosphere created by the staff. Healing is accelerated immensely when care providers can focus their intention and attention on helping patients heal.

Planetree helps organizations create patient-centric models that focus on healing and nurturing patients' bodies, minds and spirits. Currently, 319 institutions in the United States and other countries are designated Planetree facilities and have created patient-focused models that include mind, body, and spirit principles in patient care.

Now back to the reality of the American healthcare system. Most of our current facilities are far from the healing environments created in Planetree-designated hospitals or the North Hawai'i Community Hospital. Many hospitals have environments that are stressful, hurried, and chaotic instead of calm, healing, and supportive.

Much focus has been directed toward problems in healthcare in recent years. Specialization of healthcare providers has improved care within the specialty areas yet has led to an increased fragmentation in the overall care of people. Many have described the system of care today as "silos," with multiple specialists looking only at their particular aspect of care. No one is looking at the whole person's care.

To illustrate the shift in specialization, consider that in 1970, the average male had two clinicians caring for him—a primary care provider (PCP) and a dentist. The average female had three (PCP, dentist, and OB/GYN). In 2013, the average person had 15 providers—including (and not limited to) some variation of a PCP, dentist, chiropractor, OB/GYN, dermatologist, orthodontist, gastroenterologist, urologist, cardiologist, pulmonologist, rheumatologist, endocrinologist, psychiatrist, surgeon, neurologist, ophthalmologist, otolaryngologist, acupuncturist, massage therapist, nutritionist, physical therapist, fitness trainer, nephrologist, allergist, oncologist, infectious disease specialist, orthopedic surgeon, and/or plastic surgeon.

Future healthcare models must find a way to integrate care so that a person's health is evaluated within the context of whole-person care. We must move away from the silo mentality, with each provider working independently, to a model of teamwork where each discipline and specialty contributes its expertise for the benefit of the whole person.

Integrated Healthcare

The Affordable Care Act was created to help address some of these monumental issues in the healthcare system today. One component of the ACA encourages electronic health record (EHR) systems. This way, multiple healthcare providers can access the medical record, so care can be communicated, streamlined, and provided in an integrated fashion.

The Mayo Clinic is an exemplary model of an integrated healthcare system with an EHR, to which each provider contributes. Currently, under the ACA, all healthcare providers (except solo practices and practices with fewer than 10 employees) must use an electronic health record.

The intention behind this is good. However, the orchestration of converting to such systems has created multiple issues. Many patients have reported to me that they feel more attention is given to the computer in the room rather than to them. This has generated an enormous amount of frustration for providers as well. Many physicians have opted to retire and close their practices rather than compromise their integrity to deliver care focused more on an electronic record than on the patient.

We must not allow this to be the case. New electronic record systems must be proficient, concise, and helpful as opposed to another obstacle to patient care. Also, these electronic health records are not currently accessible by all providers. It appears that the onus will be on patients to communicate care from one provider to another. While this has the benefit of ensuring that people take more responsibility for their own health, it still lacks a healthcare professional evaluating the whole picture.

As we institute EHRs into hospitals and healthcare environments, we must remember that nothing enhances healing more than a caring, compassionate environment. As care providers, we must realize that patients and families are going to be anxious and fearful when their health is in jeopardy.

I certainly am not my best self when I am nervous and scared. Simply recognizing and acknowledging patients' fears can go a long way toward helping us as providers be more patient, kind, and compassionate. Focus and attention should be prioritized on developing caregivers' communication skills and helping them to enhance their sense of presence when delivering care, so that kindness and compassion predominate.

Providing a caring and compassionate attitude, especially in the emergency departments and intensive care units, is vital for patients and families. Not only are patients critically ill, but families' fears are exacerbated. Many patients and families are confronting mortality, perhaps for the first time. Fear of death and dying is recognized as one of a person's greatest fears. Imagine, day in and day out, dealing with patients and families whose loved ones are on the brink of death. These are extremely stressful and emotional environments for patients and families and for healthcare staff. Deliberate attention needs to be paid to creating compassion-focused atmospheres for patients, families, and staff.

When I think of creating positive, caring environments, I am reminded of my friend Maggie. She was a good nurse with whom I worked in the coronary care unit. At the age of 40, she was diagnosed with ovarian cancer. Her experiences as a patient, on the other side of the fence, transformed her into a great nurse. Here is Maggie's story in her own words.

Maggie

It was May 13, 1995, when my whole world changed. I'd been a registered nurse since 1987, working primarily in critical care. On this day, I became a patient; I became one of them. I learned I had ovarian cancer. That's when I realized how difficult it truly is to be on the other side of the fence. My abdomen was distended; I had pelvic pain and felt nauseated. I didn't tell the staff of radiology I was a nurse. I didn't want to intimidate them. What an eye-opener! I wish I had a nickel for every time I've been called "honey."

Guilty. I guess I should have a nickel for every time I've said it. I sat in the hall alone trying to drink barium. Suddenly I became aware that I was invisible. I listened to the staff complain about the hospital and the boss. I learned all the gossip, who's having an affair with whom, etc. I guess they thought I was deaf, but more likely I'd become less than human—a piece of meat. Guilty, guilty, guilty … Paybacks are hell.

When I went in, they smiled, explained the procedure for the CAT scan as though reading from a card. Behind the screen, they continued to socialize as though I was not there. After a while, silence; the smiles were gone; their faces blank. I knew something was terribly wrong. They said my doctor would call and he did.

Everything went quickly, and I found myself waiting for surgery—an exploratory laparotomy. I was scared to death! Again, I became a piece of meat, an object. I lost my humanity. There was a ray of light before surgery. A wonderful nurse, who held my hand, spoke to me, me the person, not the patient. She reassured me and calmed me. I'll never forget her kindness and compassion. After surgery, I awoke and as they extubated me, my abdomen was on fire. The pain was unbearable. My complaints of pain were met with annoyance and irritation. If I closed my eyes, it was assumed I was asleep. I was not. Once again, I was witness to a complaining staff and gossip. I remember every word and the indifference with which I was treated.

That was two years ago. Since that time, I've been treated very well on many occasions, but the feeling of being an object and not a human being unfortunately persists. Now I'm unable to work, but I pray for the last two years that I always treated my patients with the same kindness and compassion that the nurse I had before surgery taught me. That kindness, combined with a positive attitude, is the key to comfort and recovery.

Maggie's personal experiences with her own health challenges presented greater clarity and insight for her as to what it's like being on the other side as a patient. She continued her nursing work for two years after her diagnosis. Her delivery of care was greatly affected by her personal experiences. She would greet her patients with a smile and find a way to connect with them. She would tell each one, "Today is going to be a good day." Then she would find some reason to validate her declaration such as the patient's color was more normal, the night nurse reported that the patient slept better, his pain was less, or the lab work had improved. She would find some way to inspire the patient and give the person hope. I often observed that Maggie's patients required less pain medications and anti-anxiety drugs while she cared for them. She provided a great model for how we as nurses can deliver healing, compassionate nursing care.

Maggie died on February 17, 2003. She outlived her predicted length of life by six years. Her unfailing sense of humor was a big contributor to her longer life. Let's learn from her experiences. As caregivers, our focus must be crystal clear on the needs of the patient. No patient should be left alone in a hall trying to drink barium. All caregivers, regardless of what aspect of care they provide, should be trained to be caring and compassionate, and to be sensitive to each patient's emotional and psychological needs—especially when patients are scared and potentially receiving dreaded news about their health.

Many of my nursing colleagues still work in hospital settings. I hear frequently about their frustration and inability to practice as they have imagined. Much of their time is consumed with charting on electronic medical records or filling out standard forms that are required legally, taking valuable time away from direct patient care.

In one of our local hospitals, a recent change made to decrease costs was to eliminate respiratory therapists in the intensive care units and emergency departments. Who is expected to take over these duties? Nurses! This is on top of the tasks that already-overburdened nurses are expected to perform. This is a disaster waiting to happen, leading to an even higher degree of frustration, burnout, and risk for unsafe care. It's perplexing to me how hospital administrators could make such decisions. One lawsuit would quickly eradicate any potential savings from decreasing respiratory therapists' positions. All nurses realize this. This is clearly a "cutting off your nose to spite your face" approach.

We must create systems that allow providers to practice to the full extent of their licensure. Nurses by nature are holistic. Our basic training prepares us to look at the whole picture—body, mind, and spirit. Not only do we care for a patient's physical needs, but also psychological, emotional, and spiritual needs. We want to provide this complete care for patients. We recognize and know the importance and need for care centered on the whole person.

This improves patient care, increases patient satisfaction, and greatly enhances the satisfaction and enjoyment for nurses. This is why we chose the nursing profession: to help people through all facets of health and well-being along the entire spectrum from birth to death. Not to just chart information on an electronic record.

So how can we create ideal healing environments for patients and families? First, the design of healthcare institutions should evoke calmness and compassion. Soft colors should be chosen to promote serenity and a feeling of well-being. One hospital uses large pictures of beautiful local scenery and landscapes, strategically placed throughout the hospital. These pictures are serene, relaxing, and familiar to patients, since they are photographs taken in local parks. These images of nature from local environments nurture a sense of calmness and connectedness for patients and families. Using full-spectrum lighting provides a softer effect rather than the harsh fluorescent lighting. Every area should be designed with patient and family comfort in mind.

Compassion and caring must be paramount during patient interactions. Effective communication skills that convey compassion and concern for all patients and families should be the norm. Employees should be encouraged to go the extra mile for patients and families. This attitude of caring and compassion will reassure patients and families that the staff has their best interests in mind. Imagine if staff realized that their interactions with patients and families were literally interventions and that these interventions are just as significant as any pill or treatment.

Imagine if everyone worked together to help achieve ideal patient outcomes. In my role as a critical care specialist, I helped write outcome pathways for each of the common diagnoses of patients in the intensive care units. We met with all the team providers, including a physical therapist, occupational therapist, speech therapist, respiratory therapist, social worker, nurses, and physicians. Each professional knew his or her role for each patient's care and well-being. This was communicated to patients and families through patient care conferences in which all the care providers would meet. The entire team, along with the patient and family, created the treatment plan to achieve optimal outcomes. Everyone was on the same page and aware of the patient's health goals in order to achieve the highest good for the patient and family. This fostered a spirit of teamwork and collaboration.

Today, the care delivery system is often chaotic and fragmented— again the silos approach where practitioners are working in isolation instead of as a team. Many patients and families tell me they feel as if the left hand doesn't know or understand what the right hand is doing, leading to confusion, frustration, and dissatisfaction. Different providers and practitioners may give conflicting information regarding the patient's health status depending on the specialty these providers are evaluating, causing further frustration and confusion.

We must create a patient-centered delivery system where the needs of the patient and family are considered the utmost priority. What if the system were truly patient-centered and designed with the patient's goals as foremost? What would that look like?

A patient-centric model will place the needs of the patient and family first and foremost. Care will be prioritized to allow the patient six to eight hours of uninterrupted sleep. Morning laboratory assessments and provider rounds will be done no earlier than seven a.m. to allow the patient adequate rest. Whole healthy food will be served without using processed foods, preservatives, GMOs (genetically modified organisms), or artificial sweeteners. Therapies will be scheduled throughout the entire day and evening with rest periods in between.

A Team Approach

A team approach to patient care will be used, ensuring the best outcomes for patients and families. Each member of the team will contribute and communicate their expertise toward the patient's treatment plan with the rest of the team members so everyone (including the patient and family) is knowledgeable regarding the plan of care.

Perhaps this is achieved through patient care conferences or via a patient care coordinator who communicates with each member of the team. A summary of the patient's treatment plan could be documented on the electronic medical record with members of each discipline contributing his or her input to the overall plan so that all practitioners see the entire plan.

Everyone, including practitioners and hospital employees, who interacts with patients and families will know that her or his particular role is vital to achieving optimal outcomes for the patient. Recognition and acknowledgement that all team members are integral to achieving optimal patient care can go a long way toward fostering teamwork and a spirit of collaboration instead of competition, disregard of other staff members, or working in silos.

Caregivers will be empowered, recognized, and acknowledged for their unique contributions toward achieving patients' outcomes. This spirit of teamwork will benefit patients and create deeper satisfaction and fulfillment among caregivers.

---

1. Planetree Alliance website, https://planetree.org/, accessed October 23, 2017.

CHAPTER 3

Creating Systems that Support All Providers and Caregivers

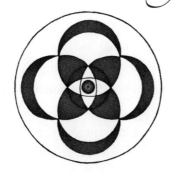

Caring and Compassion in Healthcare

Caring and compassion must take precedence not only for patients and families, but also for care providers. Dr. Robin Youngson, a physician in New Zealand, is the author of *Time to Care: How to Love your Patients and Your Job*.[1] He has challenged all healthcare providers to bring *care* back into healthcare. Interestingly, New Zealand has a national healthcare system. Dr. Youngson has never been paid one cent by a patient for care. Yet, New Zealand has similar problems in its healthcare delivery system as does the United States, including:

- An over focus on the physical aspects of care

- Disease care instead of prevention, wellness, and healthcare

- Overemphasis on biotechnology

- Unrealistic expectations for care providers, leading to staff being overloaded or overwhelmed, burned out, and experiencing compassion fatigue.

I am struck by the similarities of issues despite completely different payer sources. Apparently not all of our US healthcare problems can be blamed on economics, third-party payment (or nonpayment), health insurance infrastructure, and dominance of pharmaceutical companies. Recognizing the worldwide magnitude of the impact of the above-mentioned issues on healthcare delivery systems, Dr. Youngson created "Hearts in Healthcare," an international organization designed to rehumanize healthcare. Dr. Youngson stated, "Healthcare's focus on physical disease and biomedicine is unbalanced. We need to pay much more attention to emotional, psychological, and spiritual well-being and the huge importance of healing relationships."[2] He is committed to creating an International Center for Happiness in Healthcare to help support care providers of all professions. He has chosen Louisville, Kentucky, as the place to create the center, due in part to the citywide mission started by Mayor Greg Fischer on November 11, 2011, declaring Louisville an international city of compassion. Dr. Youngson's center will be a resource for nurturing and supporting all care providers while spurring the creation of new compassion-based models of care for both recipients and providers.

Creating new models in healthcare will require restructuring many aspects of our current system. As early as 2010, the Institute of Medicine acknowledged the pivotal role that nurses have in the transformation of healthcare in the United States. The IOM partnered with the Robert Wood Johnson Foundation and created a committee that developed an initiative outlining the future of nursing.[3] Both organizations recognized the importance of nurses, both individually and collectively, in order to transform healthcare in the United States. Their collective vision is: "The committee envisions a future system that makes quality care accessible to the diverse populations of the United States, intentionally promotes wellness and disease prevention, reliably improves health outcomes, and provides compassionate care across the lifespan."[4]

The committee established four key messages for the nursing profession:

1. Nurses should practice to the full extent of their education and training.

2. Nurses should achieve higher levels of education and training through an improved education system that promotes seamless academic progression.

3. Nurses should be full partners, with physicians and other health professionals, in redesigning healthcare in the United States.

4. Effective workforce planning and policy-making require better data collection and an improved information infrastructure.[5]

Currently some states limit the ability of advanced practice nurses to practice to the full extent of their scope of education by requiring collaborative agreements with physicians for prescriptive authority or supervised practices. Like other professional practices, such as medicine and law, nursing has its own standards of practice, educational requirements, and ethical guidelines to obtain and maintain licensure for practice. Nursing and medicine are interdependent, yet autonomous practices. To be truly patient-centered, both professions must work together, and each must be allowed to practice the full expression of their respective professions.

Reclaiming Nursing

I stated in the previous chapter that nurses, by nature, are holistic and are trained to care for people along the entire spectrum from birth to death. Yet many current systems are not conducive to nurses being truly able to practice to the full extent of their training. Imagine that you are a nurse caring for a patient who the previous day had a total mastectomy for stage four breast cancer. As you check her dressing and give her medication, she starts to cry and shares with you that she feels she is less of a woman now that her breast is removed. You know that she is hurting, grieving, and scared of what the future holds. You want to stay, to console, comfort, and explore her fears and emotions relative to all that she is experiencing. Yet you know that there are four to six other patients who need your attention. This is an all-too-familiar scenario that commonly occurs in the clinical setting.

The working climate in which many nurses find themselves is one of inadequate staffing, high patient loads, and unrealistic expectations to deliver competent and compassionate care to all the assigned patients. Not only is this type of environment unconducive for nurses to practice fully, but also this climate can lead to nurse frustration, fatigue, burnout, and powerlessness. It's easy to understand then, why nurses take on characteristics of oppressed groups, out of sheer desperation and frustration. Behaviors such as horizontal violence, "eating our young," or outward displays of negative emotions such as hatred, bitterness, frustration, anger, or jealousy emerge. The real value that nursing brings to patients and healthcare institutions is frequently invisible, or at best difficult to measure. The nurse's true value is in relating to patients, being present for them, and witnessing their pain, grief, or illness.

Here is how one of my nurse colleagues described her experience as a new nurse:

> I decided to become a nurse late in life. I was a mature student who was serious about my classes. I brought to my studies the perspective of life experiences, including the experience of past hospitalizations. The word "nurse" is a synonym for nurture, to educate. I believe in holistic nursing—caring for the whole person. I was certain nursing provided the opportunity to make a positive difference in my patients' hospital experience by providing medical care as directed in a holistic nursing care environment that nurtured the body and spirit.

> Sadly, I found the hospital setting doesn't promote holistic care. Care providers tended to their assigned body parts. Nursing assistants checked vital signs, LPNs [licensed practical nurses] tended to their designated parts, RNs [registered nurses] charted the course of care, and the patient/person was frequently lost in the process. Patient and nurse satisfaction is questionable; nursing burnout is a certainty.

Several years ago, the Joint Commission on Accreditation of Healthcare Organizations, the major credentialing organization, required that all hospitals use a pain scale to assess patient's pain and discomfort. Most people are now familiar with "Rate your pain on a scale of 0 to 10," with 0 being no pain and 10 being the most acute pain you have ever experienced in your life. Some hospitals have even used this data to help quantify the value of nursing. One obvious problem with this system is that the ideal score for nursing is zero. This is not very empowering. Also, just because a patient may not have any pain doesn't necessarily mean that his or her needs have been met. Wouldn't it be much more effective to ask patients, "How comfortable are you? What can I do to make you more comfortable?" Using the same Likert scale, now a very comfortable patient would rate a 10. This shift effectively raises the value of nursing from 0 to 10.

In October 2013, I started a mission through the Kentuckiana Holistic Nurses Association, called "I've Got Your Back" to help nurses create more positive, supportive working relationships with each other. Imagine a nurse working on a busy shift and circumstances occur beyond her or his control, such as a patient requiring more time and skill than anticipated or being assigned another admission on top of the current assignment. These scenarios are common. Usually the nurse just has to do the best that he or she can, and is left feeling inadequate, guilty, and stressed. Imagine that this unit has adopted the "I've Got Your Back" attitude. Now the other nurses step in to help, so that care can be delivered to all patients in a timely manner seamlessly, regardless of the interruptions and changes in workload. Perhaps the other nurses administer the medications, so that patient care is not interrupted by unforeseen circumstances. This is done in an atmosphere of knowing that on any given day, that same nurse might be able to "pay it forward" by providing similar assistance to her or his colleagues. This would be such a healthy environment in which to work. I've got your back!

We must also create support networks for our young nursing colleagues. Many enter nursing with some vulnerability and naïveté about the profession. Some put unreasonable expectations on themselves that may be exacerbated when more seasoned nurses treat them as if they are inadequate, uneducated, or inexperienced instead of mentoring them positively. Many new nurses leave their first position, or worse yet, leave the nursing profession entirely after the first year. We must change this. We've got to create "I've got your back" support for new nurses.

In May 2014, one of our local universities gifted their senior nurses with an afternoon designed to help them make the transition from student nurse to registered nurse. Stephanie Barnett, who is a local leader in healthcare transformation and active in the Compassionate Louisville Healthcare Community, along with nursing school professors Kathy Hager and Elizabeth Fitzgerald, created an "I've Got Your Back Day" for the graduating seniors. I presented my concept to begin the program. kRi and Hettie, a local musical duo, performed their popular song, "You Inspire Me," with a change in their beginning lyrics to, "I've got your back." Lois Luckett, a licensed clinical social worker, guided participants through a powerful experiential, meditative exercise with one person holding another's back while stating "I've got your back" three times. Next the seniors participated in a café-style group discussion to brainstorm answers to three questions:

1. How do you see yourself leading the way differently from how you've seen healthcare previously led?

2. What can you do next?

3. What tools would you need?

Each senior nurse was invited to sign an "I've got your back" pledge committing to: "Raise the value of nursing from 0 to 10 by modeling healthy behaviors and supporting all nurses and healthcare providers to be their best in body, mind, and spirit." Phone numbers and emails were exchanged, and all agreed to be available to give support and encouragement on those days or times that nursing is overwhelming or frustrating. It was a phenomenal day. I was greatly inspired by the honesty, integrity, and commitment of these nursing seniors. I believe in the future of nursing. We must continue to strengthen the profession and not weaken it.

Carrying this attitude of "I've got your back" into hospitals can inspire and support all nurses and providers so that both the patients' and staffs' needs can be met. When nurses work together as a team and know they can depend on each other to help when unexpected events occur, a cooperative supportive spirit emerges. This atmosphere fosters the acknowledgement that all team members are important and bring their own unique gifts to the service of patients. Cooperation and teamwork can generate a sense of trust, security, and an emotionally healthy environment for the staff. When this atmosphere is not fostered, the energy of a unit or hospital can become one of fear and chaos, leading to distrust and frustration among providers. It's in the best interest of all to transform the energy of the environment to one of love, compassion, trust, and caring.

Successful healthcare systems of the future must take a serious look at the conditions and obstacles caregivers must overcome to care for patients. It is not healthy and not safe for a nurse or any other professional to work 12 to 13 hours without eating or using the bathroom facilities other than a quick #1. Yet, this is commonplace in many institutions. How can nurses (or other providers) keep their composure, compassion, energy, and excellence in care if they are abusing their own basic needs? Realistic expectations of caregivers must be supported with adequate staffing, coverage for meal times, and 15-minute breaks.

Anita Tucker and Steven Spear extensively researched the obstacles, interruptions, and operational failures common for nurses working in hospital settings. Here is what their research revealed:

- One study found that nurses, on average, spend 42 minutes of each eight-hour shift resolving operational failures such as missing medications and broken or missing equipment.[6]

- Other studies showed that nurses spend 10–25 percent of their time looking for other staff members.[7]

- Tucker and Spear sampled a cross-sectional group of six US hospitals to examine the frequency of work system failures and their effect on nurse productivity. They found that nurses experienced an average of 8.4 work system failures per eight-hour shift.[8]

More recently, Rivera and Karsh analyzed 32 studies on healthcare professional interruptions in patient care. Some interruptions were necessary to safe, high-quality care, such as monitor alarms and communication on updated patient orders or information. Other interruptions were non-purposeful or operational failures that distracted the provider or prevented them from delivering optimal care. The authors suggested that when providers are doing tasks that require undivided attention, measures be taken to proactively limit interruptions to only those that are absolutely necessary.[9]

Put the Focus Back on Patients

Kathleen Bartholomew, RN, along with her husband, John Nance, authored *Charting the Course: Launching Patient-Centric Healthcare*.[10] The book chronicles the transformation of a hospital by a fictional Will Jenkins, MD, who has been recently hired as a new CEO at Las Vegas Memorial Hospital. Though written as fiction, this book is an accurate reflection of many hospital systems in the country, which operate as physician-centric or traditional biomedical models.

First Dr. Jenkins spends three weeks undercover, getting to know and understand the system for which he is about to assume leadership. He learns who the informal leaders are and the behaviors and actions of the predominant physicians. He explores every area of the hospital including the dietary department, housekeeping, operating rooms, emergency departments, and each patient care unit, by posing as a newly hired orderly. Experiencing the system directly, he arms himself with the knowledge of inefficiencies in operational methods and potential breaches in patient safety. He is also able to directly experience physicians and staff with poor communication skills. He then formally accepts his position as CEO. He rolls out his plan to move the hospital from a physician-centric model to a true patient-centric institution to the board of directors. Here are the five major tenets of his mission:

1. Create a true patient-centric institution in which everything, including finances, is subordinate to the best interests of the patient.

2. Create a physician staff dedicated to team-oriented forms of practice based on science and proven methods.

3. Create parallel bylaws for the hospital board and the medical staff with clear codes of conduct that treat everyone equally.

4. Create a proud and cohesive sense of commonality, mutual respect, and communication (vertical and horizontal) in which enthusiastic ownership (not just involvement or engagement) is to be the minimum requirement for membership.

5. Trust is to be re-established as a standard by transforming the current fear-based culture by evaluating human errors and mistakes, not as potential disciplinary occurrences,

but as important messages reflecting the underlying system, which needs to be systematically addressed.

Though these five tenets may appear simple, implementation of them would require a complete change in the culture for most hospitals and could profoundly shift any healthcare institution toward a patient-centric model. For instance, in the first tenet, Dr. Jenkins emphasizes, "everything, including finances, is subordinate to the best interests of the patient." This means that if one of the nurse managers identifies that extra nursing staff is needed to safely meet the needs of patients, she has the authority to add staff without approval from an upper-level manager. This is quite different from many hospital boards in which finances are the driving force and staffing numbers are predetermined by budgetary needs, with little regard to the fluctuation of the patient load.

The second tenet: "to create a physician staff dedicated to team-oriented forms of practice based on science and proven methods," again sounds simple. However, the reality of the implementation might not be so easy. Dr. Jenkins recognized that not every physician would embrace a team-oriented approach in which all team members were equal. Some of the seasoned physicians who were used to a physician-centric model in which physicians are viewed as superior to other providers, might be resistant to change. Dr. Jenkins planned to selectively retain only those physicians who could support the hospital's vision and commitment to a patient-centric model. He knew this would require openness on the part of the physicians to enhance relationships with other providers and be willing to change their practice patterns when research and evidence proved that such change would be beneficial to patient outcomes.

The third tenet created an infrastructure supported by the hospital board and the medical staff that emphasized respect for all team members with a zero tolerance for disruptive behaviors of any kind. As mentioned previously, traditional biomedical models run the risk of creating a culture of physician superiority or dominance. These types of systems may create an unfair balance of power among care providers in the hospital.

Some physicians have abused this balance of power by exploiting or verbally abusing nurses or other staff. This behavior should never be tolerated. It is completely disruptive to creating a healing environment, as well as unnerving to the recipient. In traditional biomedical models, this behavior is commonly met with a "turn the other cheek and ignore it" attitude.

Hospital systems that cater to physicians often have no recourse or formal policy to confront physicians' disruptive behaviors. These episodes erode other professionals' confidence and self-esteem and destroy morale. Dr. Jenkins emphasized ideal interpersonal relationships and collegial interactive teams. He supported the notion that every healthcare provider and discipline was a valuable and equal member of the team, contributing their unique expertise to the best outcomes for patients.

The fourth tenet emphasized that every employee was part of the vision and mission of the hospital to create a patient-centric model. Dr. Jenkins inspired all employees to take ownership enthusiastically and acknowledged each one for personal value and contribution toward the hospital's mission and vision. To demonstrate the equal importance of every employee, Dr. Jenkins had an open-door policy, making himself available to any employee who had an idea, suggestion, or issue. He welcomed and encouraged innovative thinking from all to help the hospital move from a disease-care model toward one of wellness and disease prevention.

The fifth tenet was profoundly important in creating a healthy, supportive culture. Dr. Jenkins engaged every employee in making patient safety a top initiative of the hospital. He encouraged employees to identify the system's potential barriers that could lead to breaches in patient safety. Most importantly, if a human error or mistake occurred in patient care delivery, information was collected and analyzed, not for disciplinary purposes, but rather to identify underlying system failures that could have contributed to the situation. This tenet reflects a true culture of "I've got your back," where all employees are working together for the best outcome for patients and families—a true patient-centric system.

Most of my colleagues (physicians and nurses) would line up to work for an institution where the best interests of the patient are paramount over everything—including finances. Dr. Jenkins's model truly is the blueprint for patient-centric hospital systems of today. Creating systems that foster patient safety with optimal outcomes based on best practices, staffing models based on patient load, collegiality among all disciplines through a team approach, and ensuring that all staff members practice to the full extent of their licensure, can radically shift the care delivered in today's healthcare institutions. Additionally, these changes can transform the culture within an organization to one that values all providers and employees equally.

Yet, current cultures in healthcare institutions are not that easy to change. Let me illustrate with an example. Dr. Peter Pronovost, a critical care specialist at Johns Hopkins Hospital, decided to create a checklist to help decrease complications from central line catheter infections. The checklist was very simple and included five steps for the physicians who were inserting the central line into patients in the intensive care unit:[11]

1. Wash hands with soap.

2. Clean the patient's skin with Chlorhexidine antiseptic.

3. Put sterile drapes over the entire patient.

4. Wear a sterile mask, hat, gown, and gloves.

5. Put a sterile dressing over the catheter site once the line has been inserted.

Though these steps are routine and appear over-simplistic, Dr. Pronovost had the nurses observe the doctors for a month before they instituted the checklist and found that in more than one third of the patients, at least one step was omitted. The next month, Dr. Pronovost persuaded the hospital administration to institute the checklist and empower nurses to stop the doctors if they observed that a step had been omitted. Fifteen months later, they realized the following results:

- The 10-day line infection rate decreased from 11 percent to zero.

- Forty-three infections and eight patient deaths were prevented.

- The hospital saved over $2 million in costs.[12]

Dr. Pronovost went on to create several other checklists for intensive care unit procedures and found them also to be extremely beneficial in improving patient outcomes.[13] He began speaking around the country about his results, but not surprisingly, he was met with enormous resistance. Many physicians felt the checklist was unnecessary and belittling and viewed it as just another bureaucratic invasion from administration.[14] They doubted that a simple checklist could yield the same results that Dr. Pronovost attained.

In 2003, the Michigan Health and Hospital Association asked Dr. Pronovost to test three of his checklists in all of the Michigan intensive care units, since their hospitals had higher-than-average infection rates. This project came to be known as the Keystone Initiative. In

December 2006, the findings were published in the *New England Journal of Medicine*. The infection rate in Michigan's ICUs decreased by 66 percent. In the first 18 months, the Michigan hospitals saved an estimated 1,500 patients and $175 million in costs.[15]

Dr. Gawande, who authored *The Checklist Manifesto*, contacted Dr. Pronovost to see why he thought there was such resistance to his idea. Here is Dr. Pronovost's response: "The fundamental problem with the quality of American medicine is that we've failed to view delivery of healthcare as a science. The tasks for medical science fall into three buckets. One is understanding disease biology. One is finding effective therapies. And one is ensuring those therapies are delivered effectively. The third bucket has been almost totally ignored by research funders, governments, and academia. It's viewed as the art of medicine. That's a mistake, a huge mistake. And from a taxpayer's perspective, it's outrageous."[16] He went on to describe that we have a National Institutes of Health that has been a great resource for discovery, but there is no National Institutes of Healthcare Delivery studying how to best incorporate these discoveries into daily practice.[17]

Yes, my colleagues, we have our work cut out for us. But I believe that we can create patient-centric models of healthcare truly grounded in evidence-based best practices and delivered with confidence and compassion. We must overcome the resistance of traditional, physician-centric, autocratic, "We've always done it that way" models of healthcare and institute best practices no matter how mundane or simplistic they might appear. Our patients and families are counting on us.

---

1. Robin Youngson, *Time to Care: How to Love Your Patients and Your Job* (New Zealand: Rebelheart Publishers, 2012).

2. Hearts in Healthcare website, https://heartsinhealthcare.com/, accessed October 23, 2017.

3. Committee on the Robert Wood Johnson Foundation Initiative on the Future of Nursing, *The Future of Nursing: Leading Change, Advancing Health* (Washington, DC: Institute of Medicine/National Academies Press, 2011), https://www.nap.edu/read/12956/chapter/1, accessed October 23, 2017.

4. Ibid.

5. Ibid.

6. Anita L. Tucker, "The Impact of Operational Failures on Hospital Nurses and Their Patients," *Journal of Operations Management* 22, no. 2 (2004): 151–69.

7. Elaine Tilka Miller, Carol Deets, and Robert V. Miller, "Nurse Call Systems: Impact on Nursing Performance," *Journal of Nursing Care Quality* 11, no. 3 (1997): 36-43.

8. Anita L. Tucker and Steven J. Spear, "Operational Failures and Interruptions in Hospital Nursing," *Health Services Research* 42 (2006): 643–62.

9. A. Joy Rivera and Ben-Tzion Karsh, "Interruptions and Distractions in Healthcare: Review and Reappraisal," *Quality and Safety in Health Care* 19, no. 4 (2010): 304–12.

10. Nance and Bartholomew, *Charting the Course.*

11. Atul Gawande, *The Checklist Manifesto: How to Get Things Right* (New York: Picador, 2011); and Atul Gawande, "The Checklist," *New Yorker Magazine: Annals of Medicine*, December 10, 2007, https://newyorker.com/magazine/2007/12/10/the-checklist.

12. Gawande, *Checklist Manifesto*; and Gawande, "The Checklist."

13. Ibid.

14. Ibid.

15. Peter Pronovost et al., "An Intervention to Decrease Catheter-Related Bloodstream Infections in the ICU," *New England Journal of Medicine* 355 (2006): 2725–32.

16. Gawande, "The Checklist."

17. Pronovost et al. "Intervention to Decrease Catheter-Related Bloodstream Infections."

CHAPTER 4

Being Your Own Patient Advocate

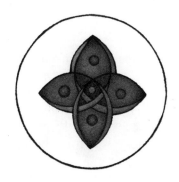

In the previous chapter, I described the culture and imbalance of power that occurs in traditional authoritarian, biomedical models. One of the underlying consequences is that when we are consumers of health, we are conditioned to seek outside expert opinions whenever anything is wrong with our body, mind, or spirit. Of course, I am not discouraging or minimizing the value in seeking professional help when needed. It can be lifesaving and greatly beneficial; however, as healthcare providers, we must not negate or overlook a person's inner knowing and intuition about their own body-mind system. Many times, patients have a good idea of what problem or dysfunction they are experiencing. As providers, we must listen to patients and encourage them to monitor their patterns and notice the subtle signs or symptoms that their body is experiencing. We must acknowledge a person's innate wisdom on what to do to help heal their body-mind complex.

Here is what I like to share with my patients: "No one knows your body, mind, and spirit better than you. That is why it's important to listen to your body. While you may seek expert opinions and advice regarding your health and well-being, ultimately your health is up to you. That's why it's so important for you to take responsibility for your own health." We must teach and encourage our patients to be their own patient advocates.

Consider Jane's story. Jane was a friend from high school. At age 35, she convinced her OB/GYN to order a mammogram due to her strong family history of breast cancer. Her paternal grandmother, aunt, and cousin had all been diagnosed with breast cancer. She asked her doctor for annual mammograms but was told that that wasn't necessary. Jane was not convinced and asked for another mammogram at age 37. Jane was told the results were similar to her mammogram done at age 35. At age 40, she discovered a lump on her breast and was scheduled to see a surgeon. In preparation for her appointment, she picked up the films of the previous two mammograms. A report from her second mammogram (done three years earlier) read: "I reviewed this individual's mammogram at age 35 and there has been significant fibrocystic change. I suggest that this individual have yearly mammograms."

Jane said, "No one ever told me that part!"

Jane's OB/GYN had not communicated this to her. Three years had passed since the radiologist's recommendation to do annual mammograms. The lump that Jane discovered turned out to be ductal breast cancer. She was subsequently treated with chemotherapy, radiation, and a mastectomy. She died about ten months later. She documented the sequence of events and asked me to please share her story so that this would not happen to anyone else. Would earlier detection and treatment have saved her life? We will never know for sure, but Jane was convinced that she might have had a different outcome that could have saved her life.

Jane's experience illustrates some of the possible gaps in communication that can occur in healthcare. Her story emphasizes just how important it is that we each take charge of our own health. We should not totally rely on our providers to get information for us or to communicate all the relevant information from lab tests and diagnostic reports. Insist on getting printed copies of all health reports including lab work, X-rays, or other tests and procedures.

Create and store your own medical file. Sometimes sequential lab tests over time may reveal subtle changes that might be relevant to your health and not be recognized with an isolated lab test. Keep your personal health file updated with all your current data. Not only will this compile a complete past health history, it could also provide vital information for continuing care by your practitioner.

It's critical to be your own advocate. This may mean standing up and confronting your physician or insurance company. Consider Karen's story. In 1998, when Karen was 32, she was diagnosed with cervical cancer. Her physician recommended a total hysterectomy, which he thought would cure her. He based this not only on her clinical presentation, but also on the very strong history of cancer in her family. She had multiple relatives who had been diagnosed with cancer and several who had died from it. However, her insurance company at the time denied her claim for the procedure, which at that time would have cost over $14,000. Instead, her insurance company informed her it would cover an alternative procedure, which involved removing only part of the cervix rather than the entire uterus. This procedure cost $787.13. Since the alternative procedure couldn't guarantee that she would be cured, she appealed the denial, only for her insurance company to deny it again.

Karen was very distraught and couldn't understand why an insurance company would deny a treatment recommended by her physician. She sought an attorney who filed a grievance against the insurance company's ruling and this too was rejected. Karen decided to go ahead with the total hysterectomy. The day before the scheduled surgery, a representative from the billing department of the hospital called, instructing her to bring $5,000 to be paid the next morning. Borrowing the money from her dad, Karen went to the hospital the next morning. The first person to meet her at six thirty in the morning was from the billing office. She told Karen that she had been assigned the task of making sure the patient would be "good for the money" before proceeding with her surgery. Karen had the surgery and ironically, the patient who shared her post-operative room had received a similar diagnosis and the same surgery. Except that in that patient's case, her insurance company covered the hysterectomy.

Karen later filed a lawsuit against Humana on the advice of both her OB/GYN and attorney. A jury sided with her and awarded $13.1 million for the case. Karen felt this was a huge victory, not only for herself, but for all those men, women, and children who had previously fought against insurers' decisions. What an example of standing up for yourself. Of course, Humana appealed the decision and it was settled out of court. Karen had only two requests for the settlement:

- That the ruling stand

- And that she clear at least $5,000 to repay the money lent to her by her father for the surgery

Learn to listen to your inner guidance. If something doesn't sound right to you, don't accept it as the gospel. For instance, if your primary care provider tells you that nothing is wrong or that nothing else can be done to help you, do not accept that as a final answer. Such a response probably means that there is not a surgical procedure or prescription medication that can be readily prescribed for your particular symptoms. These are the two main tools in a Western medicine toolbox. Or, perhaps your illness is not easily limited to one specific organ or cause.

Remember that your PCP is working for you. If you do not feel comfortable asking questions or discussing your health concerns with your PCP, choose another provider with whom you feel comfortable. Consider this story one of my patients shared.

My patient's father and stepmother had traveled to the Mayo Clinic in Rochester, Minnesota, when her father was diagnosed with a significant illness. At the first meeting with the doctor, her stepmother pulled out a tape recorder to record the visit so that they would not miss any important information. Seeing this, the physician stated that she was not comfortable with the session being recorded. Without missing a beat, the stepmother replied, "Well then, we are not comfortable having you as our doctor." Another appointment was scheduled with a different physician, the meeting was recorded, and the couple left the clinic feeling satisfied with a plan and notes that were transcribed.

It's critical that a partnership be established with your PCP in which both the provider and you as the patient feel comfortable discussing health issues. Asking providers ahead of time if they are comfortable with recording the visit might alleviate discomfort for both the provider and patient. As this story illustrated, it can be greatly beneficial to have a family member or healthcare advocate with you when you meet with your PCP, so another set of eyes and ears are present to ensure that important health information or questions do not get missed.

Here is another example of being persistent in finding the right PCP. A young woman began having symptoms of severe dizziness, nausea, vomiting, and ringing in her ears (tinnitus), which totally incapacitated her. She did a massive amount of research and found the symptoms were consistent with Meniere's disease. She went to her PCP, who told her she would just have to learn to live with it. She was dissatisfied with this response and thought there must be more that could be done. She went to another PCP. This doctor took the time to listen to her story and asked what she had learned in her research. He admitted that he didn't know a lot about Meniere's disease and said he would like to research it and have her return in one week. When she went back to see him, she discovered that he had consulted with a local expert on Meniere's disease. He shared with her what he had learned, and together they created a treatment plan, which has subsequently been quite successful.

What a difference in these two office visits. How often have you heard a health practitioner admit that they don't know something about a disease? How would you feel seeking medical advice from someone who didn't know about your disease? Yet, this doctor was able to help her significantly. I believe in some ways, we've done a disservice to healthcare providers by expecting them to know it all. This is an impossible task for any human. Approaching healthcare as a partnership between the provider and patient truly yields the most positive results as this example illustrates. Keep seeking help until you find the right provider to help you.

The current structure of healthcare (i.e., 15-minute office visits) has forced many physicians and primary care nurse practitioners into too little time to adequately evaluate patients. In many cases, the provider can only focus on one symptom or one issue. Practicing from this model, issues can be overlooked or missed when a provider does not take time to step back and look at the whole picture. Consider Debbie's story.

Debbie came to see me a few years ago for cardiovascular management. She had a previous history of breast cancer and a strong family history of heart disease. When she went to her PCP in mid-2014, her cholesterol was mildly elevated, so her doctor prescribed atorvastatin (Lipitor), which is a cholesterol-reducing drug. Normal cholesterol is below 200, LDL is below 100, and normal fasting blood sugar is below 100. Six months later, she came to see me and was very upset because even though her total cholesterol and LDL were significantly lower (134 and 39 respectively), her fasting blood sugars were rising (up to 130–140), her thyroid was stressed (indicating hypothyroidism), and her liver enzymes were elevated (liver strain). Her doctor now wanted to prescribe two additional medications—levothyroxine (Synthroid) for her thyroid and metformin (Glucophage) to help reduce her blood sugar levels.

This is clearly an example of a prescribing cascade—adding additional medications to treat side effects from the original medication, instead of trying to figure out why her chemistries were out of balance. I have long believed that there is a point at which driving the cholesterol too low can affect other organ functions (specifically liver) and alter body chemistries. I thought the reaction of her blood sugar and thyroid was complicated by the altered chemistries from the statin.

I reviewed her daily food intake and gave her a heart-healthy nutrition plan. I also recommended that she stop the atorvastatin (Lipitor). In 12 weeks, her cholesterol did increase (217 with an LDL of 130), but her thyroid, liver enzymes, and blood sugars all normalized. We created a plan to treat her cholesterol with fish oil and time-released niacin, which avoided further prescription medications that were no longer indicated.

Here is another patient, Tracy, who listened to her intuition and inner voice to direct her care. Here is her story in her own words:

Tracy

Listen. Yes, listen. Listen to your gut, listen to your inner voice, and listen to your body. I did and doing so in late November 2015 saved me. I felt like something wasn't right. Nothing really tangible, but I just didn't feel like myself. I am very social and active. I love getting out and about. Now, and for the last few months, none of that interested me. I was always tired. My stomach was bothering me. Bloating, reflux. I eliminated things from my diet. I stopped drinking . . . I know, drastic measures. Nothing helped. After a colonoscopy and endoscopy came back clean, I returned to my doctor.

I was still complaining of the same bloating and reflux symptoms; he patted me on my leg and said he thought I had IBS (irritable bowel syndrome). No, I had read about this and my intuition just said, "No, it is more than that." I told him, "No, I am not satisfied with that. I just feel like it is something more." Further tests were ordered, including a CT scan of the lower abdomen and there it was. Cancer. Renal cell carcinoma. Kidney cancer. The results came back the day before Thanksgiving. Additional doctor visits at the beginning of December confirmed kidney cancer. Thankfully, it was small and slow growing. I asked if the inevitable surgery could be postponed until after Christmas. My doctor agreed that it could be delayed.

My husband and I wanted to keep it quiet because we did not want this hanging over our children through such a beautiful time of the year. The calendar turned, and on January 6, 2016, I had surgery to remove the cancer from my right kidney. It was small, contained, and had not spread. Thank God. The morning after my surgery, the doctor came in and said I now was clear. Margins and nodes were all clear! He did tell me that the tumor was in "the worst spot possible," which was right next to the main artery leading out of my kidney. Had this not been caught, it would have likely grown into my artery and spread throughout my body, quickly.

I listened to my body and it saved my life. This cancer was found by accident. It is very rare for women to have this type of cancer, and the location within my kidney could not have been worse. I truly believe the "voice " I heard within me was God nudging me to pursue this.

I think we are not quiet enough sometimes. Our lives are full, and we find ourselves running around, having multiple distractions, phones in our faces 24/7, and we don't stop long enough to listen. I am now a member in a club I did not wish to join. This experience has changed how I look at many things, but does not, and will not hang over my head daily.

I thank God for healing me. I thank my sweet, incredibly strong husband, Frank, for waiting on me hand and foot. I thank my beautiful children for helping be my arms and legs and keeping me laughing. Lastly, I thank our family and friends. The incredible words of support, beautiful flowers, yummy food, box of sunshine, ongoing texts checking on me, and the prayers you all prayed are *so* appreciated.

So, it's done. Move on . . . but *listen*.

Sometimes we need to be advocates for our children. Here is a story from a friend of mine who describes how valuable her mother's intuition became in the healing of her infant son, Bubba.

Bubba's Story

This is our son's story [abbreviated for the purposes of this book]. Bubba was born on February 29, 2012. He weighed 6 pounds, 12 ounces and was 20 inches long. The umbilical cord was wrapped around his neck twice and he was blue and limp. I thought he was dead. My heart sank and began to race at the same time. He was not dead, but he wasn't doing well. He was having trouble breathing. After the nurses worked with him, I held him for a mere two minutes and then he was rushed to the neonatal intensive care unit (NICU). His daddy followed him, and I sat in total disbelief as to what had just happened. This is not what I imagined for my firstborn!

For the next seven days, he stayed in the NICU with breathing issues, was given multiple antibiotics for suspected sepsis (which I was not told about at the time, and only discovered when I obtained his medical records later) and had seriously high jaundice levels requiring phototherapy. On day six, he had vastly improved and was breastfeeding well. They told us we would be going home that day. We were ecstatic!

Our happiness was short-lived. Bubba received a hepatitis B shot. Within an hour or two, he was screaming as if in pain, having trouble latching for feeding, and just deteriorating in general. The nurses informed us that he would have to stay another night. I was shattered. Back then I had no idea why he deteriorated. Since then I have realized that the hepatitis B vaccination contributed to his decline that day.

We brought him home March 8, 2012. Things were better, but not for long. Each time he would nurse, he would immediately curl up in a ball and wail in pain. The pediatrician just chalked it up to colic and blew us off as overly concerned new parents. We would become quite familiar with this treatment from doctors through the next year of his life.

I knew there had to be more going on with Bubba besides colic. My mother instincts were strong, and I knew I wasn't crazy. I knew that following nursing was when he was in the most pain. This is when my journey of self-education began. I read that sometimes babies can have sensitivities through breast milk to foods the mother is eating. At this point in my life I knew nothing about food. I didn't know what preservatives or GMOs (genetically modified organisms) were and had no clue why someone would pay more money to buy organic food because I didn't know what organic even meant. I was 23 and clueless. I ate lots of bread and cheese, drank chocolate milk out of the jug, and put margarine on just about everything (I'm cringing writing this, but I believe it's an important factor in Bubba's story). I stopped eating dairy products in hopes that it would help our little guy. It worked. I was right. He began to sleep a little longer. He was happier. He seemed pretty strong.

When Bubba was two months old, we took him for his well-baby checkup, which included the following seven vaccinations all given at one time: diphtheria, tetanus, pertussis, haemophilus influenzae type B, polio, Prevnar, and Rotateq. This seemed like a lot of medications and vaccinations for one 12-pound, 12-ounce baby. Following the vaccinations, he was miserable. He screamed inconsolably and would not eat much. I was told to give him Tylenol for the fever and pain. I later learned this was just adding fuel to flame. These same vaccinations would be repeated at four and six months of age.

After each round of vaccinations, Bubba had the same reactions—inconsolable crying, decreased appetite, and fever. We naively asked his pediatrician about the safety of vaccines. We were laughed at as if we were idiots to even ask such a "dumb" question. We were assured they were completely "safe and effective" (those were really the words they used). Against our gut instincts, we continued to vaccinate.

Around eight months he started to say "dog" when he would see Charlie, our pit bull mix. Besides "Mama" and "Dada," this was his first word. At nine months, he received a second dose of the hepatitis B vaccine and a flu shot. He never said dog again. He didn't speak again besides "Mama" and "Dada" until after he was two years old. He was slow to sit up on his own and never crawled. He stared out the window for large parts of the day. He began waking in the night screaming inconsolably for one to two hours at a time. The doctors called it "night terrors" but had no explanation as to what they were or what caused them. When Bubba was 12 months old, he received the varicella vaccine.

Bubba began having ear infection after ear infection and was treated with multiple rounds of antibiotics. He had a constant runny, stuffy nose and was lethargic all the time. He began to open and close cabinet doors, bedroom doors, closet doors, and any door he could find, almost constantly. He didn't care about playing with toys: just the doors. Open. Close. Over and over, no matter how many times I redirected. It was like he was in a trance when he would do this. The night terrors went on.

He still wasn't speaking. Not a single word except one day he randomly said "tiger" plain as day after hearing it on TV. We tried to get him to repeat it, but like every other attempt to get him to speak, we had no success. He never said it again, and we could not get him to clap his hands like most other children his age. At 15 months, he received the third dose of hepatitis B, MMR (measles, mumps, rubella), and the hepatitis A vaccinations.

The ear infections continued, and we began to become more and more concerned with his lack of speech. We were assured "he'll talk when he's ready." My motherly instincts kept telling me that something was seriously wrong. We had his hearing tested to see if he couldn't hear, thinking that might have been the reason he wasn't speaking. The hearing test came back fairly normal but showed a small amount of fluid on one ear. He had tubes placed to drain the fluid and we were told they would help with the ear infections. The tubes helped with the infections, but still no speech.

Fast-forward six months: At this point, we had a newborn daughter and a sick little 21-month-old boy. After watching our daughter become constantly sick for weeks at a time after each round of vaccinations, I looked at Granola Daddy and said, "We are not going to vaccinate them anymore. This is ridiculous!" He agreed with me. We were finally beginning to trust ourselves and put all the pieces together.

Something told me to start searching for answers. I began to read about autism. Bubba had no diagnosis. I asked the pediatrician if he thought Bubba could be on the autism spectrum. He laughed and said, "Oh no, if he gives you hugs, he's not autistic." This did not seem accurate to me.

I researched until the wee hours of the morning. I found stories of families who had success with removing gluten and dairy from their child's diet. The next day we started the gluten-free, dairy-free diet. He got worse. He began having horrible tantrums where he would throw himself on the floor and scream and make noises over any and everything. He had night terrors every night for a week.

And then it all stopped. It was as if a veil was lifted. We began to see our true son for the first time. He began to attempt to speak. He said something that resembled "I love you" for the first time ever within two weeks of beginning the new diet. He didn't say it again until almost a year later, but it didn't matter to us then. It was one of the happiest moments of our lives. We knew we were on the right track. Although he was beginning to speak, we requested a referral to be evaluated for therapy to help him make progress with his speech and behaviors such as hand flapping, spinning, running into walls, tantrums, and touching everything he laid his eyes on.

At the time of the evaluation, Bubba had been on a gluten-free, dairy-free diet for two months and had been doing Epsom salt baths as a therapy we understood to detox his body. The results were astonishing. No more night terrors. Bubba continued to try some words, there was less opening and closing of doors, and he had an overall happiness and clearness that radiated from him. He was a totally different child. He was evaluated and found to qualify for both speech and occupational therapy (OT) once a week. The evaluator performed an MCHAT (Modified Checklist for Autism in Toddlers). The results were as follows: "The MCHAT screening was conducted in the home today with the parents. Child failed three items, so he is considered to be 'at risk for autism.'"

Remember that he had been on the diet for two months by this time and had shown leaps and bounds of improvement. If I would have answered those questions even a month prior, he would have definitely been considered on the autism spectrum by that test's standards. The OT concluded that he had sensory processing disorder.

We tested Bubba for food allergies due to his highly self-restricting diet. He tested positive for more sensitivities than I could even imagine. He was sensitive to cow's milk, peanuts, tomato, wheat, and many others according to the test. We had already eliminated milk and wheat-gluten with great success, so we decided to eliminate tomatoes and peanuts, as well. We followed a diet called AIP (autoimmune protocol)—a strict paleo diet. He made more strides.

Within six months of therapy, Epsom salt baths, and strict adherence to the AIP diet, he progressed from a nine-month-old speech level to beyond a three-year-old level at only two-and-a-half years old. His sensory issues were almost nonexistent. The therapists could not understand how he progressed so quickly. We shared with them what we were implementing with him. The OT shared our story with another family that had a toddler on the autism spectrum. Within a month, that child was discharged from therapy because his parents began doing what we were doing, and the child progressed rapidly. That family specifically told her to tell us, "thank you from the bottom of their hearts." I will never forget that day and how I felt. As much as our little guy suffered, something good came from it. Because of Bubba, another child was led out of the darkness.

We have continued to research optimal nutrition. In the past few months, we have transitioned to a vegan diet, 100 percent organic, non-GMO, and implemented juicing and green smoothies into our daily regimen. I believe these are the steps that are going to put us on the path to full recovery for our entire family. We have never felt better than we do currently!

As for our Bubba now, he is the sweetest boy you will ever meet. Despite all the physical and emotional pain he's been through, he has an incredible kindness that shines from within. He is everyone's friend. He is a protective big brother. He never stops talking. He speaks on a kindergarten level and is beginning to read and do math at age three and a half. Through his suffering have come awareness, knowledge, positive change, and healing.

I always say everything happens for a reason. I believe Bubba's story was written to change the world. His small fingerprint has left its mark and my greatest wish is that his story will continue to inspire, educate, and spread truth.

My friend's story is compelling and triggers emotional reactions on many levels. The field of vaccination safety is fiercely debated and for many is highly controversial. The American Academy of Pediatrics will defend vaccinations and say that they are safe and effective, have helped to eradicate communicable diseases, and are in no way connected to the autism epidemic. Yet, Dr. Ginger Taylor has documented 142 research papers that support that vaccinations may be a causative factor in autism.[1] If you speak with parents of children like my friend, there was an obvious decline in both of her children's health after each round of vaccinations. From her experience, this mother now believes that all vaccinations are bad. This is not good from a public health perspective. The pediatrician did not take the time to listen to her fears, and the parents did not feel as if they had a voice in how to best care for their children.

I clearly understand the public health benefits of eradicating communicable diseases with vaccinations. However, as healthcare providers, we must take a closer look at the use, safety, timing, and efficacy of vaccinations. Future research must focus on why some children tolerate vaccinations while others clearly have adverse reactions. Did all the antibiotics that Bubba received during his first week of life disrupt the microbiota of his infant gastrointestinal tract, predisposing him to intestinal permeability and immune dysfunction? Should his immune system have been given time to recover before injecting the hepatitis B vaccination? Does a newborn infant who is a few hours old really need a vaccination for hepatitis B if the mother has never had hepatitis? Are we giving too many vaccinations? Are we administering too many vaccinations at one time? Does an infant truly need a flu vaccination? These are questions that beg further investigation.

Thimerosal (diethyl mercury) is a common preservative that was previously used in many vaccinations. Research has shown that thimerosal can induce significant cellular toxicity in human neuron and fetal cells, leading to neurodevelopment disorders such as those seen in the autism spectrum.[2] Thimerisol has been removed from all vaccinations except the flu vaccine since 2010. However, the incidence of autism has not decreased.[3]

The preservative that is used most commonly now is aluminum. Researchers have found that aluminum may also be implicated in neurological diseases.[4] Evidence is also showing that people who have a specific genotype may have more difficulty metabolizing and clearing metals such as mercury or aluminum.[5]

The gene is the APO E gene. There are three alleles of the APO E gene—2, 3, and 4. Each person receives one APO E allele from each parent, resulting in one of six possible combinations. The 3/3 APO E gene is the most common, occurring in 60 percent of the population.[6] Continuing research is supporting evidence of a higher incidence of complications from vaccinations in babies who have an atypical genotype, especially when they carry the 4 allele.[7] Only 22–27 percent of the population has a 4/3 APO E and fewer than 5–7 percent have the 4/4 APO E.[8] Over 70 percent of children do not carry a 4/3 or 4/4 genotype and might conceivably be unaffected by the aluminum in vaccinations. Could this account for the reason that research associating vaccinations to autism is inconclusive? I certainly think it is a possibility.

Edward McDonagh, DO, founder of the McDonagh Medical Center in Kansas City, reports that a physician in North Carolina, Dr. Buttar, tested 15 children who developed autism after their vaccinations. All 15 carried the 4/4 APO E. The webpage where I first found this study has since been taken down. Communications with the author, Rashid Buttar, DO, have gone unanswered, possibly because of the repressive stance Big Pharma has taken against anyone questioning vaccine safety. That stance is also parroted by public health officials, who seem to be under their influence. My colleague Pam McDonald has also noted a much larger percentage of ADD, ADHD, and autism in children who have an APO E of 4/3 or 4/4.

Perhaps in the future, a baby's APO E gene will be tested at birth. If the child has a variant APO E (4/3 or 4/4), then perhaps a reduced vaccination schedule would be followed or perhaps some vaccinations might be omitted for these infants. As healthcare providers, we need to expand our thinking and acknowledge that the current vaccination schedule and practice may not be safe for everyone. While it is very difficult to accomplish given the highly politicized attacks on those questioning vaccine safety, further research on vaccination efficacy must be carried out so that future clinical decisions can be guided by unbiased evidenced-based data. This is certainly not the case now.

Let's explore another area that requires you to be your own advocate, which is understanding your health insurance coverage.

Insurance practices are changing daily. Most people do not know what their insurance company will and will not cover.

This is critical information for you to understand. For every healthcare service in which you use your health insurance, you will receive an Explanation of Benefits (EOB). Make sure that you understand how to read your EOB. These are not bills. They are only explanations of how your medical claims were processed. The subsequent bill will come directly from the provider of the service such as your physician or nurse practitioner's office or the lab that did the tests that were ordered for you. It is very important to match the EOB to the actual bill to prevent overpayment. The insurance companies will list codes on the side to explain how your benefits were applied.

In many cases, insurance companies will not cover a test unless there is sufficient medical necessity. For instance, when my husband had his labs evaluated for his annual examination, he had an advanced lipid panel to determine his cardiovascular risk. Part of this panel includes testing the homocysteine level, which had been elevated on his previous blood tests. The insurance company required the medical records to determine the medical necessity of this test. This took several months and several phone conversations to reprocess the claim. On the original invoice, the homocysteine level was billed at $178.54, which the insurance company would not cover. Once his medical record was submitted to them, documenting the medical necessity, the claim was refiled, and the amount that we were responsible for decreased to $13.

In summary, you are your best advocate to create your optimal health and well-being. Here are the necessary steps to being your own patient advocate:

- Keep your own medical file, including records of all provider office visits, all laboratory reports, X-rays, surgeries, or other tests and procedures. All patients are entitled to one free copy of their medical records.

- Find a provider who will be a partner in your care and that you are comfortable asking questions of. You may want to explore using an integrative medicine provider who will look at the whole picture of your health and well-being—body, mind, and spirit.

- Never hesitate to get a second opinion if you don't feel comfortable with your health assessment and plan from your PCP.

- Do your own health research and do not rely on your provider to give you all the information you need on creating your optimal health.

- Understand your healthcare benefits and how to interpret your EOBs.

- Never pay a healthcare-related bill unless it matches your EOB.

---

1. Ginger Taylor, "142 Research Papers Supporting Vaccine/Autism Causation," SCRIBD website, https://www.scribd.com/doc/220807175/150-Research-Papers-Supporting-the-Vaccine-Autism-Link, accessed October 23, 2017.

2. David A. Geier, Paul G. King, and Mark R. Geier, "Mitochondrial Dysfunction, Impaired Oxidative-Reduction Activity, Degeneration, and Death in Human Neuronal and Fetal Cells Induced by Low-Level Exposure to Thimerosal and Other Metal Compounds," *Toxicological and Environmental Chemistry* 91, no. 3–4 (2009): 735–49; and Boyd E. Haley and Teri Small, "Interview with Dr. Boyd E. Haley: Biomarkers Supporting Mercury Toxicity as the Major Exacerbator of Neurological Illness, Recent Evidence via the Urinary Porphyrin Tests," *Medical Veritas* 3 (2006): 921–34.

3. Centers for Disease Control and Prevention, "Vaccine Safety. Thimerosal in Vaccines," CDC website, https://www.cdc.gov/vaccinesafety/concerns/thimerosal/, accessed October 23, 2017.

4. Lucija Tomljenovic and C. Shaw, "Aluminum Vaccine Adjuvants: Are They Safe?" *Current Medicinal Chemistry* 18 (2011): 2630–37; and Christopher A. Shaw et al., "Aluminum-Induced Entropy in Biological Systems: Implications for Neurological Disease," *Journal of Toxicology* (2014), http://dx.doi.org/10.1155/2014/491316.

5. M. E. Godfrey, D. P. Wojcik, and C. A. Krone, "Apolipoprotein E Genotyping as a Potential Biomarker for Mercury Neurotoxicity," *Journal of Alzheimer's Disease* 5, no. 3 (June 2003): 189–95, http://www.optimalfunctioning.com/research/godfrey-et-al-2003-apolipoprotein-e-genotyping-as-potential-biomarker-for-mercury-neurotoxicity.html; and Robin Bernhoft and Rashid Buttar, "Autism: A Multi-System Oxidative and Inflammatory Disorder," *Townsend Letter* (April 2008).

6. Pamela McDonald, APO E Gene website, https://apoegenediet.com/.

7. Ibid.

8. Ibid.

CHAPTER 5

Integrative Medicine: A New Paradigm for Practice

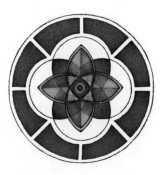

*It is much more important to know what sort of patient
has a disease than what sort of disease a patient has.*
—Hippocrates

For us to transform healthcare, we must make a profound shift from
our current disease models of care to a model of wellness and disease
prevention. Many integrative medicine providers are changing
the paradigm of medicine. Here's a definition for integrative

medicine from the website of the University of Arizona Center for Integrative Medicine: "Integrative medicine (IM) [is a] healing-oriented medicine that takes account of the whole person (body, mind, and spirit), including all aspects of lifestyle. It emphasizes the therapeutic relationship and makes use of all appropriate therapies, both conventional and alternative."[1]

The subtle difference Hippocrates notes (in the above quote) illuminates the fact that each person is unique. One's body chemistry, emotions, and experiences make a significant difference in how an illness may manifest. Disease does not occur in the same manner, frequency, or intensity for everyone. Integrative medicine acknowledges individuality and the unique experience of each patient. There are eight major tenets of an integrative, holistic practice.[2] Let's take a brief look at each one.

1. Partnership between patient and practitioner

This is an integral part of integrative medicine. Patients are partners in their care. No one knows his or her body better. As an integrative medicine provider, when I present a treatment plan to a patient, we discuss it. If the patient has any resistance about any part of the plan, we discuss the patient's hesitation, reasoning, and then modify the plan until there is mutual agreement on how the patient can best meet health goals. This is not always the case in the current biomedical model. My patients often tell me that their primary care provider (PCP) gave them a prescription for a medication, but that the patient decided not to take it for one reason or another. In many cases, the providers have no idea that their patients did not follow their recommendations. The current biomedical model does not afford time or infrastructure for a dialogue to occur to establish mutually agreed-upon health goals.

2. Appropriate use of conventional and alternative methods to facilitate the body's innate healing process

In my integrative medicine practice, I use a wide array of therapies and other practitioners to help patients achieve their optimal health of mind, body, and spirit. Since stress contributes to or exacerbates many processes of disease in the body, I employ several stress management tools. One such tool is Amma Therapy, an acupressure approach based on traditional Chinese medicine. It involves muscle manipulation, massage, and pressure points along the 12 major Chinese meridians. Many of these meridians are associated with an emotion. For instance, the lung channel holds onto grief; the kidneys, fear; the liver, anger; and the gall bladder, frustration, resentment, and bitter disappointment. Not only is Amma Therapy extremely beneficial for stress reduction, it also helps to move the energy of unprocessed emotions from the body. Amma Therapy is effective for pain reduction. Chronic pain patients need non-pharmacologic options to reduce or eliminate pain. Bodywork such as Amma Therapy, massage, Healing Touch, Jin Shin Jyutsu, and chiropractic care fall into this category.

I employ many methods of breathing exercises to help patients manage their stress and increase their well-being. One of my favorite breathing techniques is Dr. Andrew Weil's 4-7-8 breathing technique. Dr. Weil contends that if you do four breath cycles of this technique twice a day (eight breaths total), for 30 days, then your parasympathetic nervous system (the calm, relaxed part of your nervous system) will be dominant over the sympathetic nervous system (the fight-or-flight, high adrenaline part of your nervous system). Wouldn't you like the calm, relaxed part of your nervous system to be your default way of being instead of feeling stressed and anxious most of the time? And as Dr. Weil says, "This is right under your nose." Here is the simple technique:

4-7-8 Relaxing Breath Exercise
Courtesy of Andrew Weil, MD and www.DrWeil.com, all rights reserved.

1. Exhale completely through your mouth, making a whoosh sound.

2. Close your mouth and inhale quietly through your nose to a mental count of four.

3. Hold your breath for a count of seven.

4. Exhale completely through your mouth, making a whoosh sound to a count of eight.

This is one breath cycle. Now inhale again and repeat the cycle three more times for a total of four breaths.[3]

My colleague Kimberly May is certified in HeartMath® biofeedback. She is masterful at helping people learn HeartMath® to enhance parasympathetic dominance over the familiar fight-or-flight adrenaline response.

Achieving parasympathetic dominance with HeartMath® has been useful to help patients lower their stress response and their blood pressure, and to increase their happiness and joy. Kimberly is also licensed as a health coach, and she helps people set intentions and achieve goals to experience a deep sense of meaning and purpose in their lives. People find greater happiness and joy and reduce their response to stress.

Other practitioners in our integrative medicine office offer a variety of other therapies and energy modalities including yoga, massage, Healing Touch, Reiki, craniosacral therapy, Indigo biofeedback, Advanced Integrative Therapy, Yamuna Body Rolling, and the Feldenkrais Method. Each of these therapies is greatly effective in reducing the stress response, decreasing pain, and promoting relaxation and overall well-being. Our collective intention is to create a patient-centered model in which patients can achieve their optimal health and well-being. Acknowledging that each patient is unique, we offer a variety of skilled practitioners and effective modalities that patients can explore to create and enhance their individual wellness plans.[4]

3. Consideration of all factors that influence health, wellness, and disease, including body, mind, emotions, spirit, and community

Much of the focus of conventional medicine is on the physical nature of disease, with little attention to psychological, emotional, or spiritual aspects of health and well-being. Yet, nothing happens to a person physically that doesn't affect him psychologically and emotionally. And in many instances, a person may have underlying psychological and emotional issues that present as a physical complaint.

I treated a patient a few years ago with left-sided shoulder pain. He denied any strain, overuse, or trauma to his shoulder. He had full range of motion in his left shoulder but just had a continual, nagging pain. I treated him with Amma Therapy using pressure points, acupressure, and massage. I mentioned that the left side of the body frequently holds emotions related to feminine issues. He then shared that he was in the process of an intense divorce and that his ex-wife was "driving him crazy."

I explored further what he was doing to help process his feelings and emotions. He had begun to see a counselor who was helping him work through his grief, disappointment, fear, and anger. We discussed the impact on his young children and the implications for him of shared custody. I taught him the 4-7-8 breathing technique to help him manage his stress response and emotions. At the end of the visit, he was pain-free and felt confident about the plan we established for him to continue working on his psychological and emotional stressors.

I often thought that if he had sought treatment from a conventional medicine practitioner, he probably would have been treated with a steroid injection in his left shoulder. I doubt that there would have been any time to discuss his personal life. If by chance the patient had mentioned that he was going through an intense divorce, he probably would have been given a prescription for an antidepressant. An injection and prescription might have helped him over the short term but would not have provided long-term support for helping him manage the shoulder pain and underlying grief.

Integrative medicine acknowledges the influence of all of these factors—physical, mental, emotional, spiritual, and community—on one's health and well-being.

4. A philosophy that neither rejects conventional medicine nor accepts alternative therapies uncritically

Throughout my integrative medicine training, I was taught to have an open-minded skepticism, whether considering conventional medicine or alternative medicine. As integrative medicine providers, we use the same standards for research and clinical application for integrative therapies that we do for conventional therapies. Two issues make this a bit problematic.

First there is an undertone of bias in conventional medicine to use only those therapies that have been taught in medical schools. Since many alternative or integrative therapies are not taught in most medical schools, providers are reluctant to use or recommend treatments with which they are not familiar. (In fact, the classic definition for "alternative therapies" is those therapies not taught in conventional medical schools.)

I prefer the term integrative since "alternative" implies an either/ or dichotomy (conventional vs. alternative). As integrative medicine providers, we use what is deemed appropriate for the given situation. Obviously, if a patient called complaining of chest pain, I would not suggest they come to the integrative medicine office; I would tell them to call 911 immediately or hightail it to the closest emergency department. Then, once the acute emergency was managed, integrative medicine might be ideal for nutrition counseling, stress reduction, or risk factor modification.

Secondly, when medical institutions vie for research dollars, most of the money goes toward developing new pharmaceutical agents or technological advances instead of integrative therapies. Research is costly and competitive. Therapies that are non-invasive, or have a low level of risk, often are not going to be allocated research funding.

To address this issue, the federal government created the National Center for Complementary and Integrative Health (NCCIH) in 1991. Its mission is to define, through rigorous scientific investigation, the usefulness and safety of complementary and integrative health interventions and their roles in improving health and healthcare.[5] Currently NCCIH research priorities include (but are not limited to) investigations of the impact of complementary health modalities in alleviating chronic pain syndromes and inflammatory processes, and in improving health and wellness. Specifically, the NCCIH is interested in studies that will define endpoints meaningful to improved health, well-being, and quality of life.[6]

Integrative medicine practitioners focus on patient outcomes. If a therapy has a low level of risk and a high potential for having a positive outcome for the patient, that therapy will be implemented, and the patient's response will be monitored. This holds true whether or not the therapy is considered conventional or integrative. Compared to conventional therapies, many integrative therapies are cost effective with a low level of side effects.

For instance, there are many nutraceuticals—herbs and supplements that can be used in place of prescription medications—that are a fraction of the cost of pharmaceuticals and generally have fewer side effects.[7] One example is using red yeast rice for cholesterol reduction; it can be purchased as a supplement, instead of the expensive statin prescriptions. Red yeast rice contains monacolin, a chemical that lowers cholesterol and is similar in structure to some statins. Research has demonstrated the efficacy of red yeast rice in lowering cholesterol.[8] In my practice, I have found fewer side effects with red yeast rice than with statin prescription medications.

It is very important to note that in 1994, the US Congress passed the Dietary Supplement Health and Education Act, which created a new regulatory framework for herbs, nutraceuticals, and supplements. Since then, manufacturers of supplement products are now responsible for determining product safety and any label claims made about their products must be substantiated by adequate evidence. Thus, FDA approval is not needed before products are marketed. As a result, thousands of nutraceutical, herbal, and supplement companies have emerged since 1994. There is great variation among companies regarding standards of manufacturing practices and evidence of their products' efficacy. In my practice, I use only products made by those companies that are industry leaders, provide studies on the efficacy of their products, and/or who sell their products only to licensed healthcare professionals. If you are going to use herbs, nutraceuticals, and supplements, please do so under the care of a healthcare practitioner who is knowledgeable about them.

5. Recognition that good medicine should be based in good science, be inquiry driven, and be open to new paradigms

Good medicine must be grounded in good science. Studies and inquiries must have sound scientific methodologies with integrity, and results must be reported without bias or manipulation of the raw data. Many drug studies are conducted by employees of the pharmaceutical companies that manufacture the drug.

How can we be certain that no bias exists in the results when the company that makes the drug is conducting or supporting the research? As clinicians, we must be educated on sound scientific methodologies. We must attend educational conferences and keep current on scientific discoveries that affect our practices. We must not rely solely on drug representatives for current clinical information and expect it to be unbiased.

As new information is discovered, we must be open-minded and change some of our previous ways of practicing. Fifteen years ago, the American Heart Association concluded that eating eggs could increase your blood cholesterol and recommended that everyone limit the number of eggs they eat. However, further research concluded that consuming dietary cholesterol, such as eggs, does not increase a person's blood cholesterol nearly as significantly as consuming trans fats (hydrogenated oils). Newer dietary guidelines for heart health do not include an egg restriction. As providers, we must stay abreast of current research and the implications on our individual practices.

Clinical research shows that chiropractic therapy, physical therapy, massage, and acupuncture are effective modalities for patients with low back pain.[9] These measures can be just as effective in reducing pain as surgical procedures. Since these therapies are less costly and non-invasive, they certainly should be employed first. Yet, in many cases, we see that patients with low back pain are treated primarily with surgery and medications such as muscle relaxers, opioids, or narcotics. While pharmaceuticals may be warranted for short-term symptom management, they do not get to the root of the problem and are not a great strategy for long-term use. Furthermore, many of these pharmaceutical substances are addictive, which can lead to enormous long-term problems.

For us to transform healthcare, we must think of creating new paradigms such as multidisciplinary clinics that utilize all disciplines working as a team. Imagine a new paradigm for patients with back and other musculoskeletal pain. Imagine a center where chiropractors, acupuncturists, massage therapists, energy workers, surgeons, pain management physicians, and nurse practitioners work together to help patients with acute and chronic pain.

6. Use of natural, effective, less-invasive interventions whenever possible

With the continued accelerating costs of prescription medications, we must explore less expensive options. The financial burden that Americans are assuming with prescription medications is becoming unmanageable. I have had patients tell me they had to make the difficult choice of paying for their prescriptions or purchasing food. This is unacceptable. I recently saw a patient who was discovered by another provider to have a high homocysteine level and a vitamin B deficiency. The patient had a genetic mutation in the methylenetetrahydrofolate reductase gene (the MTHFR gene). A defect in this gene interferes with the multi-step process in the body that converts the amino acid homocysteine to methionine, which is necessary for making other proteins in the body. The treatment is typically to give the patient B vitamins.

This patient was given a prescription for Deplin, which is a methylated form of folate (one of the B vitamins). The retail cost of this prescription was $130 per month. For most patients, it is more effective to give a B complex that includes all the B vitamins. Integrative Therapeutics, one of the supplement companies that we use, has an Active B complex that not only has the methylated folic acid as included in the Deplin, but also has all the other beneficial B vitamins. Since B vitamins work synergistically in many of the body processes, there is value in giving all the B vitamins instead of just methylated folic acid. The retail cost of the Active B complex is $18.20 per month.

Quite commonly, a supplement or vitamin is available that is much less costly, has fewer side effects, and is generally better tolerated than the prescription drug counterpart. Yet most physicians will automatically prescribe the prescription drug first. Most medical and nursing school curricula do not include education on botanical medicine or nutritional supplements. Thus, many prescribers are unaware of botanical or supplement options that could be used safely instead of pharmaceuticals. The NCCIH has information on its website that shows the current research of many herbs and botanicals.[10]

This is coupled with the fact that pharmaceutical companies spend more than twice as much money on marketing and promotion of products ($71 billion) than they do on research and development ($32 billion).[11]

As previously mentioned, it is best to use supplements, herbs, or nutraceuticals under the direction of a licensed healthcare provider who is knowledgeable about them.

7. Focus on promoting health and preventing illness

The Centers for Disease Control and Prevention has reported that seven of the top 10 causes of death in 2010 were chronic diseases.[12] These diseases are largely preventable.

Lifestyle factors, including obesity, smoking, lack of physical activity, poor dietary habits, and unmanaged stress responses can all influence the development of chronic illness. Integrative medicine providers are trained to address each of these factors. In the next chapter, I'll include several examples of lifestyle modifications that prevent the occurrence of chronic diseases.

8. Practitioners trained to be models of health and healing, and committed to the process of self-exploration and self-development

As an integrative medicine practitioner, I learned that healing myself is an important lifelong aspect of integrative medicine. I never stop learning and exploring ways to commit to my own health. I make a conscious effort to practice what I preach and model healthy behaviors. I follow my specific APO E Gene Diet (more on this in the next chapters) and avoid wheat, gluten, and dairy, after I had tests to verify that I was sensitive to these proteins. I begin most days with a combination of yoga, meditation, and breathing exercises.

I exercise with the guidance of a fitness trainer weekly and add walking, tennis, or biking the rest of the week. I have a facial and craniosacral treatment every few months and a pedicure and maintenance chiropractic every three to four weeks. My husband and I attend our neighborhood church regularly.

I feel blessed to enjoy excellent health and know that my behaviors and actions certainly affect my well-being. Even so, I still have my own challenging patterns and behaviors. I know that I could benefit from sleeping longer and going to bed earlier than I do. This remains one of my health goals.

I love my work, and at the same time, can easily become consumed by it, so I find I must intentionally balance my work, family, friends, and leisure time. I do better at some times than others. I strive to be a model of health and healing and am committed to continuing my own journey of optimal wellness and self-discovery.

-----

1. Center for Integrative Medicine, University of Arizona, "What is Integrative Medicine?" Center for Integrative Medicine website, https://integrativemedicine. arizona.edu/about/definition.html, accessed October 23, 2017.

2. Ibid.

3. Center for Integrative Medicine, "What is Integrative Medicine?"; and Andrew Weil, "Three Breathing Exercises and Techniques," Dr. Weil's website, "https://www.drweil.com/health-wellness/body-mind-spirit/stress-anxiety/breathing-three-exercises/, accessed October 23, 2017.

4. For detailed descriptions of each of these therapies, visit integrativemedicine4u.com.

5. National Center for Complementary and Integrative Health, "NCCIH Facts at a Glance and Mission," NCCIH website, https://nccih.nih.gov/about/ataglance, accessed October 23, 2017.

6. National Center for Complementary and Integrative Health, "Research Results," NCCIH website, https://nccih.nih.gov/research/results, accessed October 23, 2017.

7. Weil, *Why Our Health Matters*.

8. Matthew Klimek, Shan Wang, and Adeleye Ogunkanmi, "Safety and Efficacy of Red Yeast Rice *(Monascus purpureus)* as an Alternative Therapy for Hyperlipemia," *Pharmacy & Therapuetics* 34, no. 6 (2009): 313–27; Maaike C. Gerards et al., "Traditional Chinese Lipid-Lowering Agent Red Yeast Rice Results in Significant LDL Reduction but Safety Is Uncertain: A Systematic Review and Meta-Analysis," *Atherosclerosis* 240, no. 2 (June 2015): 415–23.

9. Gert Bronfort et al., "Evidence-Informed Management of Chronic Low Back Pain with Spinal Manipulation and Mobilization," *Spine Journal* 8, no. 1 (2008): 213–25; John M. Mayer, Vert Mooney, and Simon Dagenais, "Evidence-Informed Management of Chronic Low Back Pain with Chronic Lumbar Extensor Strengthening Exercises," *Spine Journal* 8, no. 1 (2008): 96–113; Marta Imamura et al., "Evidence-Informed Management of Chronic Low Back Pain with Massage," *Spine Journal* 8, no. 1 (2008): 121–33; Carlo Ammendolia et al., "Evidence-Informed Management of Chronic Low Back Pain with Needle Acupuncture," *Spine Journal* 8, no. 1 (2008): 160–72; and "Acupuncture: Does It Work? For Which Indications?" *The Medical Letter* 48, no. 1234 (2006): 38–39.

10. National Center for Complementary and Integrative Health, "Herbs at a Glance," NCCIH website, https://nccih.nih.gov/health/herbsataglance.htm, accessed October 23, 2017.

11. Marcia Angell, *The Truth About Drug Companies: How They Deceive Us and What to Do About It* (New York: Random House, 2005).

12. Centers for Disease Control and Prevention, "Leading Causes of Death and Numbers of Deaths, by Sex, Race, and Hispanic Origin: United States, 1980 and 2014 (Table 19)," in *Health, United States, 2015*, CDC website, https://www.cdc.gov/nchs/data/hus/hus15.pdf#019, accessed October 23, 2017.

CHAPTER 6

Shifting to True Healthcare:
Preventive Integrative Medicine

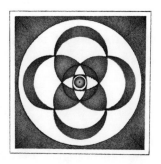

As a nurse, I was taught that health is the absence of disease. What does that really mean? This is a very narrow description of health, and if you think of health as being on a continuum, this definition makes very little sense. It implies that health is limited to an absence of physical maladies only. The current disease-oriented model certainly supports this narrow view of health. It's interesting to note that the World Health Organization in 1946 defined health as a state of complete physical, mental, and social well-being and not merely the absence of disease or infirmity.[1] Despite the fact that this definition was written over 70 years ago, providers today still mainly practice in a disease-care model where health is generally accepted as the absence of disease.

People don't typically seek medical attention until they are ill, and then an attempt is made to treat their illness. This disease-care model works well with an acute illness, accident, or injury; however, it falls very short in chronic disease states, since many chronic illnesses are hard to treat, but can easily be prevented. As providers, why do we want to wait until someone gets ill and then try to treat them? Why do we not place a greater focus on wellness and disease prevention? Especially after learning the following statistics, published by the CDC in 2015:[2]

- As of 2012, about half of all adults in the United States (117 million people) had one or more chronic health conditions. One of four adults had two or more chronic health conditions.[3]

- Seven of the top 10 causes of death in 2010 were chronic diseases.[4]

- Heart disease and cancer together accounted for nearly 48 percent of all deaths.[5]

While research also has shown that the deaths from 30 percent of all cancers, and nearly 30 percent of heart disease and stroke are preventable in the United States, only 5 percent of all research funding is spent on preventing disease.[6] Doesn't it seem logical that we can save millions of lives (and billions of healthcare dollars) if we focused on disease prevention instead of waiting for a person to become ill? One objective of the Affordable Care Act was to include more focus and coverage for disease prevention. So far, our biomedical systems remain heavily focused on disease care. For Medicare patients, prevention coverage has been limited to one wellness visit per year and limited screening tests.

Disease care is rooted in reductionism: breaking everything down to smaller and smaller parts until we find a root cause. We have believed that properties and behaviors of the parts determine the whole. For example, we have assumed that if we could just find that one biochemical alteration (or gene) that causes cancer, we could cure it. Discoveries in quantum physics, however, have turned this view on its head. We now understand that the whole is much more than the sum of its parts.

The whole also defines the behavior of the parts. In other words, the internal environment of a body influenced by physical, psychological, emotional, spiritual, and energetic factors will influence whether cancer proliferates or not. The realization that systems are integrated wholes and cannot be understood simply by the analysis of smaller and smaller parts, has shattered conventional beliefs. It appears that reductionist scientific concepts and theories are then limited.[7] It is now clear that the more we learn, the more questions we have. Because science is limited, absolute certainty is an illusion. Some concepts of health and well-being transcend science. Let me illustrate with an example.

As nurses, many of us have witnessed patients who healed against all medical odds. There were no scientific explanations. We chalked it up to the miraculous, to Divine intervention. Quantum physics and the transcendence of the mind and body open whole new possibilities. Previously we believed that consciousness was a function of only the brain. We now know, because of near-death experiences, validated by empirical evidence, that consciousness exists outside the body-mind complex, even when the body and mind are incapacitated.[8]

The phenomenon of consciousness beyond the body and mind is well documented in fascinating books such as *Heaven is for Real*,

Proof of Heaven, Dying to Be Me, and *90 Minutes in Heaven.*[9] These stories describe people who were terminally ill, unconscious, or pronounced dead. Each of them vividly recalled an experience of existence outside of their body-mind complex and articulated these experiences once they returned to this physical existence.

In chapter 1, I described Dr. Dossey's Era III Medicine, based on quantum physics and the non-local nature of consciousness. Near-death experiences are great examples of this non-local nature of consciousness. Clearly our essence is more than just the body or the mind. Imagine what is possible in healing if we transcend the body and the mind and consciously recognize the divine spiritual essence in each of us. This essence is our access to miracles. Instead of miraculous healings, seemingly occurring by chance, we can intentionally manifest such healings. Not only is this possible, it is probable, and is well documented by authors such as Gregg Braden and Bruce Lipton.[10]

Let's explore the body, mind, and spirit from the perspective of quantum physics. Quantum physics supports the fact that everything is energy. Everything has its own frequency or vibration. This is most easily depicted in Dr. Ginger Bowler's Energy Model.[11]

Imagine this list as a continuum of energy. Everything above the line is a faster, higher frequency vibration. Everything below the line is a slower, denser energetic vibration. The top of the scale is God (Absolute, Higher Power, Perfect Divine Essence)—the source of all that is, and which permeates each and every one of us.

It's impossible for us to be disconnected from God, since this is the essence from which we came into existence. Yet, sometimes, we forget or move away from God to the lower levels of vibration. You can easily recognize that everything above the line has a higher vibration, and improves our health of body, mind, and spirit. Everything below the line leads to dis-ease, disharmony, or unhealthiness.

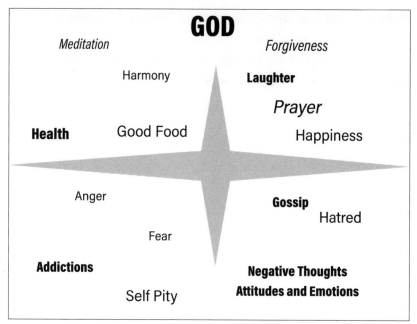

Used with permission from Ginger Bowler, PhD, ThD

Whatever energy frequency you exude attracts a similar vibrational frequency back toward yourself. This is what is commonly known as the Law of Attraction. This helps explain why it is so important to keep a positive attitude, monitor your self-talk and pay attention to what you are putting into your body energetically with food or drink so you keep your vibration high and keep yourself healthy. Frustration, negativity, and low vibration frequencies breed more of the same. Think of the phrase "getting up on the wrong side of the bed." On such a day, everything seems to go wrong. From the energy model perspective, this describes being "below the line." In the next chapter, I'll describe further how to raise your vibration physically, psychologically/emotionally, and spiritually.

Optimal health is a manifestation of all three components— body, mind, and spirit—not just the body. Alterations in any of these three areas can and do affect our overall health. Not only do I want to have an absence of disease, I want to create vibrant health and wellness. I want to have the energy to play with my grandchildren, travel, continue my integrative medicine practice, be happy, love and appreciate my family, feel connected to God, and know that I am a spiritual being having a human experience.[12] I want to live my purpose and fulfill my divine destiny.

So, you see, creating exceptional health must go beyond only the absence of disease, and physical issues. Exceptional health must include optimal well-being of the body, mind, and spirit. This is the focus of integrative medicine—to look at the whole person from a physical, psychological/emotional, and spiritual perspective.

Here are a few patient stories to demonstrate how I use an integrative model in my holistic approach to patient care. First, the patient is a partner in his or her care, and together we create a treatment plan that is practical and reasonable to follow. I see many people who have a family history of high cholesterol or heart disease. We use the apolipoprotein E (APO E) gene diet to help guide patients in reducing their risk of developing heart disease.

The APO E Gene

The APO E gene was discovered in the early 1970s. On DNA chromosome 19, the APO E gene was identified and found to come in three variations: 2, 3, or 4. Each person gets one of these gene types from their mother and one from their father, resulting in six different genotype possibilities: 2/2, 2/3, 2/4, 3/3, 4/3, or 4/4. The most common genotype is 3/3.

Each genotype is associated with different protein structures, which require different combinations of fuel sources. The 2 gene type is associated with cysteine-based proteins. The APOE 4 gene type is associated with arginine-based proteins. Cysteine types process nutrients quickly and are best supported by long-term food sources (healthy fats) while arginine is best supported with short-term food sources (healthy carbohydrates).

People who have a 4 gene in their genotype have a difficult time clearing fats and cholesterol, so their metabolism is best supported by a low-fat diet. Those who have a 2 gene are best supported by a moderate or higher fat diet.

These differing protein structures and related preferred fuel sources explain why one diet does not fit all. Everyone's metabolism is different, based on their APO E gene, thus their preferred fuel sources and diet recommendations will vary. Here are the recommended diet and exercise prescriptions based on APO E genotypes:

APO E	Nutritional Recommendations	Optimal Exercise
2/2	35% fat, 15% protein, 50% carbs	45% strength/flexibility 55% aerobic
2/3	30% fat, 15% protein, 55% carbs	45% strength/flexibility 55% aerobic
2/4	25% fat, 20% protein, 55% carbs	50% strength/flexibility 50% aerobic
3/3	25% fat, 20% protein, 55% carbs	50% strength/flexibility 50% aerobic
4/3	20% fat, 25% protein, 55% carbs	25% strength/flexibility 75% aerobic
4/4	20% fat, 25% protein, 55% carbs	25% strength/flexibility 75% aerobic

Pam McDonald, FNP, author of *The Perfect Gene Diet*, eloquently explained the science behind the APO E gene.[13] In her work with thousands of patients, she has found that when people follow a diet based on their APO E genotype, they do much better physiologically. Even those with a genetic predisposition for cardiovascular disease, diabetes, arthritis, or other inflammatory diseases who follow the recommended diet and exercise programs, do not exhibit these inherited genetic predispositions.

In other words, it's not just about genetics. The environment you put with your genetics (what you eat and drink and how you exercise), determines whether or not disease will develop based on what genes are turned off or on.

Here is a description of one of my patient's recent successes.

Charlie

Charlie is a 49-year-old father of two preteen girls who works hard to balance his life as father, husband, and main financial support for his family. Despite his stressful job, which requires many out-of-town trips per month, he creates time to be with his daughters and support their activities. In his initial visit, he revealed that he was volunteering as a soccer coach for his daughters' team. He described his lifestyle as hectic and admitted that most meals were eaten away from home at fast food restaurants. His diet history revealed consumption of mostly processed foods. The results of his initial labs were drastically abnormal. He was at severe risk of developing plaque in his arteries that could likely cause a stroke or heart attack.

I counseled him on nutrition using the APO E Gene Diet and encouraged him to eliminate fast foods, processed foods, and refined carbohydrates. I gave him a menu plan to follow and asked him to keep a daily food log. Additionally, we discussed healthy options for when he traveled out of town. I supplied a meter for him to measure his blood sugar levels to help determine which foods best supported his genotype. His supplement regimen included fish oil, Glycemic Manager, Coratin (red yeast rice), time-released niacin, and raw nattokinase. He also used a daily multivitamin for men and a probiotic. Sixteen weeks later, his repeat labs showed significant improvement. His progress was especially remarkable considering that the Thanksgiving holiday fell within the 16 weeks. This was all achieved with diet, exercise, and supplements.

Over the 20 years that I've had my private practice, I have seen many patients present with autoimmune diseases such as fibromyalgia, Hashimoto's thyroiditis, rheumatoid arthritis, interstitial cystitis, or polycystic ovaries. I have found that many autoimmune conditions begin in the gastrointestinal tract. Bear with me as I explain the pathophysiologic process.

There are millions of tiny finger-like projections called villi that line the inside of the 21-foot-long small intestine. These villi are lined with epithelial cells that help protect the gastrointestinal tract from bacteria, endotoxins, parasites, and other microorganisms. The villi have cellular structures called "tight junctions" that allow nutrients to be absorbed, but prevent toxins, microbes, or undigested food from crossing into the bloodstream. The toxins, microbes, and undigested food move on through to the large intestine to be excreted.

An intact intestinal barrier is critical to normal physiologic function and disease prevention. Probiotics and fermented foods help keep the intestinal microbes (microbiota) healthy and protected. If the intestinal barrier becomes compromised, then antigens—

the foreign molecules of invader cells and foreign molecules of undigested proteins and lipids—can leak into the submucosal tissue of the small intestine and eventually into the bloodstream.

This syndrome is called "leaky gut" or intestinal permeability. When these cells leak into the bloodstream, an inflammatory response is activated. Immune cells will identify these antigens and produce cytokines and antibodies to destroy them. Sometimes the antibodies destroy the normal healthy tissues that have similar properties to these invader antigens. This is an autoimmune disease—when antibodies are created that destroy normal healthy tissue.

For instance, if the antigens happen to be similar to the molecules of cells of the thyroid gland, then thyroid antibodies may be produced, and these can adversely affect your thyroid function. If the cells mimic those in your joints, antibodies might be produced causing rheumatoid arthritis. In my practice, I have seen that many autoimmune illnesses such as polycystic ovaries, multiple sclerosis, Guillain-Barré syndrome, psoriasis, and eczema are affected by this intestinal permeability (leaky gut) process. Undigested proteins from wheat, gluten, dairy, corn, soy, rice, or potatoes that have leaked into the bloodstream can trigger production of antibodies. The treatment priority is to heal the gastrointestinal tract, so the integrity of the villi and tight junctions can be restored. Thus, the inflammatory responses and subsequent triggering of antigens, which are causing the antibodies to be produced, can be stopped.

In our practice, we use a special lab to measure antibody production. This lab measures antibodies through the immunoglobulin A (IgA) or G (IgG) pathway. This is different from common allergy testing, which measures the immunoglobulin E (IgE) response, the immunoglobulins commonly associated with anaphylactic allergic responses. While people may not have an obvious allergy to a particular food (an IgE-mediated response causing an anaphylactic reaction), they may still have significant sensitivity to a food producing an IgG or IgA inflammatory response. People who are sensitive to wheat or gluten will develop wheat agglutinin IgG or IgA antibodies, indicating a leaky gut. IgG and IgA antibody production can result in low-level inflammatory changes in the GI tract that can cause issues such as increased gas (flatulence), bloating, abdominal pain or discomfort, diarrhea, or constipation.

I have found that 70–72 percent of the patients we've tested are sensitive to wheat and gluten. I had a difficult time understanding why so many patients reacted to wheat and gluten when Americans have been eating bread and wheat products for decades. How could this be? Something had to have changed. As I researched further, I found that most wheat is sprayed with pesticides (specifically glyphosate or Roundup) two days to two weeks before it is harvested. This practice of spraying glyphosate on wheat before harvest is known as desiccating.[14] Farmers often had trouble getting wheat and barley to dry evenly so they came up with the idea to kill the crop with glyphosate one to two weeks before harvesting to accelerate the drying of the grain. This practice has been particularly adopted in areas that have more moisture such as the upper Midwestern states (including North Dakota, which is the leading wheat-producing state in the United States).

Today, most conventionally grown crops of oats, flax, triticale, and wheat are all desiccated with glyphosate. This is despite the fact that California has recently proposed to classify glyphosate as a carcinogen.[15] A growing body of research is documenting health concerns related to glyphosate as an endocrine disruptor that affects normal estrogen and androgen function.[16] Research also indicates that glyphosate kills beneficial gut bacteria, damages the DNA in human embryonic, placental, and umbilical cord cells, and is linked to birth defects and reproductive problems in laboratory animals.[17]

Glyphosate has been used commercially in agriculture practices since 1997.[18] Could it be that glyphosate or other pesticides are the culprit of so many reactions to wheat and gluten? Despite insistence from the biotech companies that pesticides are safe and do not react with humans, evidence is showing that these pesticides (especially glyphosate) may certainly be interacting with the microbiota in the small intestine, upsetting the normal flora, and setting up the potential for intestinal permeability and an inflammatory cascade response.[19]

The following are two case studies from my practice.

Ann Marie

Ann Marie is a 72-year-old vibrant woman who has followed a holistic lifestyle for much of her adult life. She came to my office about six years ago and her labs revealed a mildly elevated cholesterol level, so I checked her APO E and advanced lipid panel to evaluate her cardiovascular risk. She has managed her cholesterol quite well with diet, exercise, and fish oil. She struggled with mild hypothyroidism and had been treated previously by a former primary care provider with thyroid hormone replacement. I checked her full thyroid panel. My suspicion was confirmed that she had elevated thyroid antibodies, which is consistent with Hashimoto's thyroiditis. This is an autoimmune condition in which the immune system creates antibodies against the thyroid gland. Eventually, this may negatively affect the thyroid function. Normally, the thyroid antibody level should be less than 34 IU/mL. Her thyroid antibodies were 91.

I encouraged her to avoid all wheat and gluten. She also agreed to use digestive enzymes and a potent probiotic. She was under enormous stress as her husband, who was 18 years her senior, had been diagnosed with an aggressive lung cancer.

Increased stress produces adrenaline and cortisol, negatively affecting the intestinal microbiota. In addition to diet recommendations and supplements, I referred her to my colleague Kimberly May for HeartMath® biofeedback to help her manage her grief, stress, and emotions. On her follow-up lab tests, after implementing the recommendations for eight weeks, her thyroid antibodies decreased to 26 IU/mL. What an improvement!

Al

Al is a 36-year-old man who presented with a 15-year history of chronic fatigue syndrome. Even as a teenager, he was very fatigued most of the time. In his 20s, he was also diagnosed with depression. He was treated with every antidepressant and combinations of medications without success. Not surprisingly, he told me he had suffered most of his life with gastrointestinal disorders of bloating, gas, nausea, and stomach pain. He added that he had been taking proton pump inhibitors for acid reflux for more than 20 years and was currently on 40 milligrams of Omeprazole daily. He felt lousy most days, suffering from persistent headaches, abdominal pain, and a severe lack of energy.

I tested him for antibodies and found that he was sensitive to wheat, gluten (rye, barley, spelt, and kamut), carrots, spinach, apples, red and white wine, peaches, nectarines, scallops, and shrimp. He eliminated these trigger foods and took a course of anti-inflammatory supplements, clinical nutrients, and a high-dose probiotic to help heal his GI tract. Within three months, Al made remarkable progress. He had no further headaches and stated he felt more energetic than he had in the previous 10 years. He was able to wean off two antidepressant medications that he had been taking for five years. His next goal was to wean off the Omeprazole, which he successfully did three months later.

Another common group of patients that I see are women with perimenopausal and postmenopausal issues. I have learned by seeing these women that there is a connection between estrogen and cholesterol levels. As estrogen begins to decline, cholesterol levels (especially the LDL—bad cholesterol) commonly increase. The good cholesterol (HDL) decreases. Many of these women are then prescribed statin drug therapy to help lower their cholesterol levels. Statins can cause stomach issues, interfering with digestion, which commonly presents as gastro-esophageal reflux. Commonly a proton pump inhibitor (PPI) is prescribed for the heartburn symptoms. While a PPI may manage the symptoms temporarily, they do not heal the underlying issue of improper digestion. Hydrochloric acid must be produced in order to digest food completely. If undigested food remains in the stomach, it putrefies, producing cadaverine, putrescine, and methane, as well as causing reflux. Proton pump inhibitors cut the production of hydrochloric acid by 90 percent, further compromising digestion. Proton pump inhibitors are recommended for short-term use only (three weeks). Yet many patients are prescribed these medications for several years. Over time, PPIs can deplete magnesium and calcium in the body, leading to further physical problems.

Estrogen levels also interact with neurotransmitters and brain chemistry. Many peri- and postmenopausal women describe feeling as if they have lost a bit of their zest for life. If they communicate this to their primary care provider, a common response is yet a third prescription medication, an antidepressant. Menopause is a natural and inevitable change in a woman's life cycle, which can be significantly supported with integrative medicine.

Following the APO E Gene Diet can certainly mitigate any potential increase in cholesterol levels. A regular exercise program can naturally increase endorphins, which may prevent the feeling of a decreased zest for life. Using bio-identical hormone replacement can minimize menopausal symptoms such as hot flashes, insomnia, vaginal dryness, or vaginal atrophy. Here is a recent patient example.

Mary Jo

When Mary Jo first came to see me, she was 58, had a mildly elevated cholesterol level, and was suffering with night sweats, insomnia, and significant hot flashes several times a day. At night, she usually required two fans directly on her just to get comfortable enough to sleep. She had been prescribed a statin by her previous provider but stopped taking this due to side effects of unbearable leg cramps. I measured an advanced lipid panel to get more detailed information about the risk of her cholesterol profile and determined her cholesterol could be managed with the APO E diet, exercise, and fish oil. A test that measures plaque in the carotid arteries verified my treatment plan, as she had minimal plaque. I started her on a low dose of bio-identical hormone replacement, which reduced her hot flashes more than 90 percent. Her improved sleep helped increase her energy level. Together we discussed stress management strategies and how to bring more joy into her life.

She began a regular yoga practice and explored other self-care techniques such as massage, Amma therapy, meditation, and HeartMath® biofeedback. She is excited about her progress in only five months.

I can share many other success stories of patients who benefited from integrative medicine and a holistic approach of body, mind, and spirit. It truly is the model and the framework our healthcare system needs to create individualized approaches for health, wellness, and disease prevention. While prescription medications and surgery are necessary, and at times lifesaving modalities, they should not be considered the only tools in a provider's toolbox. Here is another patient's story in her own words to illustrate this point.

Joy

My consultations with IIM [Institute for Integrative Medicine] practitioners Kim Evans, Jerry Scott, and Peter Buecker, MD, have been life changing. As a recently retired biologist and first responder, I have experienced life's peaks and valleys from both community and personal perspectives. I know life is a gift. A life well lived is the legacy I earnestly desire. Attaining this life goal, however, was becoming a major challenge until I became a patient at IIM. My cellular self was increasingly screaming at me via muscle and joint pain, gastrointestinal upsets, and nagging headaches, along with self-doubt about my future endeavors. My ultimate smackdown occurred while doing stable chores when I was kicked by my beloved filly. My sense of vulnerability was overwhelming. Traditional medical care was not helping me achieve the quality of life I wanted.

Thus, I confess, I approached IIM out of desperation and frustration. Kim identified my persistent GI episodes as leaky gut and lab results revealed I have several food sensitivities. Now, selective organic food is my medicine. Genotype analysis revealed sugar is my primary toxin!

No more processed food either! Goodbye brownies, donuts, and Reese's Cups! Biofeedback results by Jerry Scott confirmed that my endocrine system is out of balance. Welcome hormones! YEA! Mindful meditation taught by Dr. Pete has awakened within me a cellular self-awareness that has promoted healing and self-care while infusing new energy into my every step and thought. Physical therapy, light therapy, and physical conditioning have complemented my successful recovery on my journey to wellness. Returning to my stable duties from a 10-day absence, my filly was repentant and gave me her lovey-dovey greeting which is a soft nuzzle on my heart. A thoughtful hieroglyphic pronouncement on the stable message board presented me a soulful reminder of the ultimate healing force: love—first as self-love and, secondly, as shared love. Thank you to Kim, Jerry, Pete, Vicki, Jon, Sherri, Debbie, and Ashley. I am very awake and quite mindful!

Sometimes an integrative approach to wellness means navigating both conventional and integrative medicine. Consider Rita. I encouraged her to have an annual women's health exam since she had not had one in a couple of years. On the visit with her women's health nurse practitioner, she was found to have a lump on her right breast and was later diagnosed with stage III triple-negative breast cancer. Over the following several months, she was treated with chemotherapy, a lumpectomy, and radiation therapy. Her follow-up pharmaceutical regime pushed her into early menopause. I helped her manage her hot flashes and other hormonal symptoms with non-estrogenic supplements. I helped her create a diet based on her APO E genotype and prescribed supplements to help reduce her inflammation. All through her course of treatment, I continued to see Rita to help with her psychological support, stress management, Amma therapy, and optimal nutrition. She is now five years out from her breast cancer diagnosis. Rita states that the most significant contribution from integrative medicine was to help support her body so she could handle the toxicities of the chemotherapy and radiation treatments. She continues to follow the APO E Gene Diet and exercise program, and she uses Amma therapy and nutritional supplements to support her health.

Conventional medicine is predominantly focused on pharmaceuticals and surgical procedures. But that does not mean that other systems of medicine are not effective or important. For instance, I worked with a patient who had severe lower back pain. She had done physical therapy, but her pain persisted. The orthopedic surgeon told her that her only option was surgery. She did not want surgery unless there were no other options. She explored acupuncture and decided it was worth trying for her pain control before deciding on surgery. She had five acupuncture treatments, which completely relieved her pain. Now, 15 years later, she remains pain-free and did not have to undergo spinal surgery.

Using an integrative approach to wellness means keeping an open mind toward other traditions and modalities of healing and making use of all appropriate therapies whether conventional or alternative. I hope this chapter has illustrated, for you, the benefits of an integrative medicine approach to wellness and disease prevention.

---

1. World Health Organization, Constitution as Adopted by the International Health

Conference, New York, June 19–22, 1946, WHO website, http://www.who.int/about/mission/en/, accessed October 23, 2017.

2. Centers for Disease Control and Prevention, "Chronic Disease Overview," CDC website, https://www.cdc.gov/chronicdisease/overview/index.htm, accessed October 23, 2017.

3. CDC, "Chronic Disease Overview"; and Brian W. Ward, Jeannine S. Schiller, and Richard A. Goodman, "Multiple Chronic Conditions among US Adults: A 2012 Update," *Preventing Chronic Disease* 11 (2014): 130389.

4. CDC, "Chronic Disease Overview."

5. Ibid.

6. Marjorie McCullough, "Preventing Cancer with Food: Magic Bullets vs. Dietary Patterns," presented at the 7th Annual Nutrition and Health Conference, May 11, 2010, Atlanta, GA, file:///C:/Users/Susan/AppData/Local/Temp/NHC2010-online_brochure.pdf, accessed October 23, 2017; and Centers for Disease Control and Prevention, "Preventable Deaths from Heart Disease and Stroke," CDC website, https://www.cdc.gov/vitalsigns/HeartDisease-Stroke/index.html, accessed October 23, 2017.

7. Kimberly A. Evans (Genevieve Bartol and Nancy F. Courts, original authors), "The Psychophysiology of Body-Mind Healing," in *Core Curriculum for Holistic Nursing*, 2nd ed., edited by Mary Helming et al. (Burlington, MA: Jones & Bartlett, 2014).

8. Dossey and Keegan, "Nursing: Integral, Integrative, and Holistic."

9. Todd Burpo with Lynn Vincent, *Heaven Is for Real* (Nashville, TN: HIFR Ministries, 2011); Eben Alexander, *Proof of Heaven: A Neurosurgeon's Journey into the Afterlife* (New York: Simon & Schuster, 2012); Anita Moorjani, *Dying to Be Me: My Journey from Cancer, to Near Death, to True Healing* (Carlsbad, CA: Hay House, 2012); and Don Piper with Cecil Murphey, *90 Minutes in Heaven: A True Story of Death and Life* (Grand Rapids, MI: Revell, 2004).

10. Gregg Braden, *The Divine Matrix: Bridging Time, Space, Miracles, and Belief* (Carlsbad, CA: Hay House, 2007); and Bruce Lipton, *The Biology of Belief: Unleashing the Power of Consciousness, Matter, and Miracles* (Carlsbad, CA: Hay House, 2007).

11. Ginger Bowler, *Listening and Communicating with Energy* (Madison, WI: Focus on the Light Publishing, 2000).

12. Wayne W. Dyer, *There's a Spiritual Solution to Every Problem* (Carlsbad, CA: Hay House, 2002).

13. Pamela McDonald, *The Perfect Gene Diet* (Carlsbad, CA: Hay House, 2010).

14. Ken Rosenboro, "Why Is Glyphosate Sprayed on Crops Right Before Harvest?" Eco Watch website, March 6, 2016, https://www.ecowatch.com/why-is-glyphosate-sprayed-on-crops-right-before-harvest-1882187755.html, accessed October 23, 2017.

15. Ibid.

16. Céline Gasnier et al., "Glyphosate-Based Herbicides Are Toxic and Endocrine Disruptors in Human Cell Lines," *Toxicology* 262, no. 3 (August 21, 2009): 184–91; and Anthony Samsel and Stephanie Seneff, "Glyphosate's Suppression of Cytochrome P450 Enzymes and Amino Acid Biosynthesis by the Gut Microbiome: Pathways to Modern Diseases," *Entropy* 15, no. 4 (2013): 1416–63.

17. Gasnier et al., "Glyphosate-Based Herbicides"; and Samsel and Seneff, "Glyphosate's Suppression of Cytochrome P450 Enzymes."

18. Rosenboro, "Why Is Glyphosate Sprayed on Crops?"

19. Samsel and Seneff, "Glyphosate's Suppression of Cytochrome P450 Enzymes."

CHAPTER 7

Self-Care: Modeling and Creating Healthy Behaviors

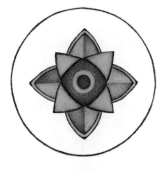

As healthcare providers, it's critical that we "walk the talk" and "talk the walk" of modeling healthy behaviors for our patients and for each other. Remember Dr. Bowler's Energy Model? Staying above the line raises our vibration, which helps keep us healthy. Let's now look at how to raise our vibration physically, psychologically/emotionally, and spiritually so we can create optimal health of mind, body, and spirit.

Raising Your Vibration of Optimal Physical Health

Here are the critical factors to creating your optimal physical health:

- Adequate hydration

- A healthy diet

- Restful sleep

- Exercise

Let me share the important aspects of each one.

Adequate Hydration

When you were born, your body was about 75 percent water. As you age, this percentage decreases. For most of us, water makes up more than two-thirds of our weight. In the elderly, hydration may be as low as 50 percent. Dehydration, especially of the brain, has been cited as a possible contributing factor of Alzheimer's disease and dementia.[1] As we age, proper hydration is critically important for other bodily systems as well, including circulatory, gastrointestinal, and muscular-skeletal health.

The water we drink should have a neutral pH of about 7. However, in many of our cities, the tap water has been shown to be acidic. Acidic water causes deleterious effects on our gastrointestinal tracts. Some bottled waters such as Mountain Valley Spring Water are alkaline (pH 7.8). Additionally, Mountain Valley Spring Water comes in glass bottles, including 2.5 and five-gallon water cooler bottles that can be reused at your home or office. Providing a glass container has the added advantage of avoiding bisphenol, a chemical found in plastic bottles.

The amount of water to drink per day continues to be debated. A familiar recommendation is to drink eight eight-ounce glasses of water daily, but this is not based on any hard science. The Institute of Medicine recommends 2.7 liters (about 91 ounces) daily for female adults in moderate climates and 3.7 liters (125 ounces) for adult men. This total includes both fluids that you drink, and the moisture taken in with foods that are eaten (usually about 20 percent of your fluid intake).[2]

I've commonly heard practitioners recommend the formula of drinking half of your weight in ounces per day of water. If you weigh 150 pounds, then at least 75 ounces of water are suggested. Obviously, water intake should be increased with warmer climates, intense exercise, and medical conditions such as fever. Generally, if you heed your thirst sensation and drink when you are thirsty, this will guide your body's need for water. Beware that the thirst sensation decreases with age.[3] Monitoring the color of your urine can be helpful to know if you are adequately hydrated. Drink water until your urine is clear or the color of pale straw.[4]

On the topic of hydration, it is worth giving attention to other beverages we might consume. Avoid soda or carbonated soft drinks. These drinks contain phosphorus, which leaches calcium out of your bones. Soft drink consumption is a huge contributor to osteoporosis in our country. Pure carbonated water does not have this effect because there's no phosphorus from added flavorings.

Remember that alcohol and caffeine cause diuresis, which means you lose excess fluid from your body. You may lose more fluid from your body than what you consume when drinking caffeinated and alcoholic beverages. This can lead to dehydration. To avoid dehydration, it's best to limit alcohol and caffeinated beverages. Green teas are excellent because most are much lower in caffeine than coffee or are naturally decaffeinated, and they include antioxidants that help support your immune system.

Healthy Diets

Nutrition has been the subject of much debate in our country and rightly so. The connection between diet and health is undeniable, but what is the healthiest diet? Much of our understanding of what a healthy diet should include has changed over the last 45 years. For instance, in the mid-1980s, the American Heart Association recognized that 45 percent of Americans were overweight, and that heart disease was a leading cause of death. To improve the health of Americans, the heart association encouraged people to consume less saturated fat, which was believed to contribute to increased levels of LDL (low density lipoprotein), i.e., the bad cholesterol. High levels of LDL correlate with an increased risk of heart disease. Food manufacturers rushed to lower the saturated fat content.

Unfortunately, much of the saturated fats were replaced with either sugar or partially hydrogenated oils (trans fats), which we now understand are more detrimental to our cholesterol levels and heart health than saturated fats. In the mid-1990s, we began to realize this mistake of replacing saturated fats with sugar or trans fats, as now 65 percent of Americans are overweight or obese, and heart disease continues to be the #1 killer of Americans.

Recently, it seems that carbohydrates—especially grains and starches—have been demonized as contributing to the obesity epidemic. Diets such as the Paleolithic or Atkins recommend significantly restricting some or most carbohydrates. The truth of the matter is that all three macronutrients—proteins, fats, and carbohydrates—are important for a healthy well-balanced diet. How much of each macronutrient and what type is again the subject of much debate. Clearly a wide range of healthy and unhealthy options exists within each macronutrient category.

In the last chapter, I introduced Pam McDonald's groundbreaking work with the APO E Gene Diet. This diet provides a commonsense approach to healthy nutrition.[5] Working with thousands of patients,

Pam has demonstrated that when a person follows a diet and exercise program based on their genetics, their health and cholesterol levels improve. Their risk for heart disease, Alzheimer's, diabetes, stroke, and other chronic inflammatory illnesses significantly decreases. Remember that there are three APO E gene variations: 2, 3, or 4. You receive one from each parent, so each of us has one of these six APO E combinations: 2/2, 2/3, 3/3, 4/2, 4/3, or 4/4.

Each genotype has a preferred fuel source, which is why one diet does not fit all. APO E gene testing can be done by blood or a cheek swab by contacting our office or Pam's.[6] Once you know your genotype, you can follow a diet with specific daily quantities of healthy servings of fats, carbohydrates, and proteins to help you achieve the recommended percentages of each macronutrient. Whether or not you know your genotype, start by choosing healthy options for each macronutrient.

Carbohydrates

Carbohydrates are necessary to give us quick energy and are thus considered a short-term fuel source. Carbohydrates include grains, starches, potatoes, pasta, fruits, and vegetables. They generally cause a rise in blood sugar significantly more than fats and proteins. See the food nutrient diagram.

The glycemic index was established to show how much a particular food affects blood sugar. It uses a scale of 0–100 with higher values given to foods that cause the most rapid rise in blood sugar. A glycemic index of 55 or below is considered low and over 70 is high. Healthy carbohydrates are generally those that are low or moderate on the glycemic index. The glycemic index has been further refined to include the amount or serving size of foods consumed. This is known as the glycemic load. Glycemic loads of 10 or less are considered low and above 20 is high. Let's look at an example to appreciate the value of the glycemic load versus the glycemic index.

Watermelon has a glycemic index of 72, which is considered high, but chances are, you are not going to eat the entire watermelon. When you look at the glycemic load based on an average serving size of one cup, the glycemic load is eight, which is low.[7]

The quickest way to determine if a product has a high glycemic index is to read the ingredients. If the product list includes high fructose corn syrup as one of the first five ingredients, it is likely to have a high glycemic index and perhaps a high glycemic load. Examples of healthy grains with low or moderate glycemic loads are oatmeal, quinoa, and multi-grain bread. Foods that are described as "enriched" are best avoided. This is commonly seen on various types of bread, and it just means that the bread has been processed to the point that valuable B vitamins have been lost. These vitamins are added back in and then the bread is advertised as enriched. Healthy starches include brown rice, sweet potatoes, and whole grain pasta. Fresh fruits and vegetables are always highly encouraged.

How Quickly Macronutrients Change Blood Glucose

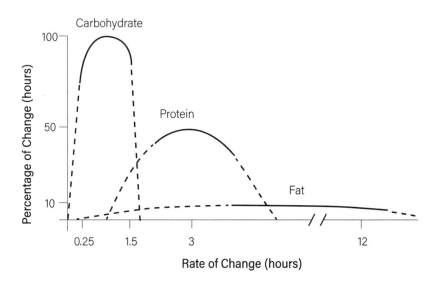

Proteins

Culturally, we have been conditioned to revere protein. Think of your holiday meals. Thanksgiving would not be complete without the traditional turkey or ham. Yet we don't need as much protein—especially animal protein—as most Americans consume.

In the CDC Dietary Guidelines for 2015–2020, the recommended daily protein consumption is 5.5-ounce-equivalents per day (not per meal). Based on a 2,000 calorie per day food plan, the recommended weekly consumption of meats, poultry, and eggs is 38.5 ounce-equivalents.[8] An average size serving of organic chicken or turkey is about 3.5 ounces. If you went to a restaurant and ordered a 3.5-ounce steak, you might feel cheated. It's not uncommon to see an order for a 16-ounce steak. This would be 62 percent of your weekly recommended meat consumption in one meal. Additionally, roughly 50 percent of animal protein is saturated fat. This steak could have as much as 16 grams of saturated fat, which far exceeds the daily recommended saturated fat intake of no more than 10–15 grams for the entire day. However, as of this writing, the thinking on saturated fats is changing, so this number may be considered too low in the near future.

Regardless, remember that not all fats are created equally, so choose them carefully—especially those in animal protein. Look for animal protein sources that are grass fed with no hormones and no antibiotics. It is worth paying a little extra for organic beef especially, because data continues to reveal negative health effects from conventional farming practices. For instance, there is 42 percent more growth hormone found in a 3-ounce serving of hormone-supplemented cattle versus non-hormone-supplemented beef.[9] Increased occurrences of reproductive cancers and early puberty development for girls are being investigated as possible consequences of the hormone-supplemented cattle.[10]

In the 1970s, the top five beef packers controlled about 25 percent of the market. Today, the top four control more than 80 percent of the market. Educate yourself. Watch the movie *Food, Inc.* to see the impact these meat producers are having on our food source, economy, and natural resources.[11] Use organic chicken or turkey. White meat has less saturated fat than the dark poultry meat. Think about eating fish for your protein. Wild Alaskan salmon, Alaskan black cod, halibut, scallops, sea bass, trout, lobster, tuna, mackerel, sardines, shrimp, and herring are all great sources of fish protein. Be leery of farm-raised seafood and fisheries that do not follow sustainable practice guidelines. Instead, choose seafood from fisheries that are certified sustainable or considered sustainable by experts such as the Monterey Bay Aquarium Seafood Watch Program. Vital Choice is one company that demonstrates high integrity in its fishing practices and offers some of the best seafood that I've ever tasted.[12]

Most of us naturally think of protein as only provided from an animal source. However, keep in mind that there are many plant-based sources of protein. All types of beans (black, navy, pinto, white, soy, and edamame) are wonderful sources of protein. Legumes such as lentils and peas have robust amounts of protein. Health risks decrease when you follow a plant-based diet.[13] The film documentary, *Forks over Knives*, based on a book by the same name, highlights Drs. Caldwell Esselstyn and T. Colin Campbell's 30 years of research proving the health benefits of plant-based diets.[14] They have demonstrated the reduction of cancer and heart disease when following a plant-based diet.

It's helpful to remember that some foods such as almonds, walnuts, cashews, and peanuts, which we consider to be healthy fats, provide excellent protein as well. Another protein-rich food typically thought of as a grain or starch is quinoa, which has 8.1 grams of protein per cup. In summary, there are many wonderful nutritious sources of protein besides that from animals.

Fats

There are four types of fats: monounsaturated, polyunsaturated, saturated, and trans fats. Two are good, one was thought to not be as good, but the thinking is changing, and one is really, really bad.

Good Fats

- Monounsaturated fats are the simplest fats. As long as they are unprocessed, they are healthy fuel sources for the body. Monounsaturated fats include olives, olive oil, avocados, palm fruit, and peanut oil. Canola oil is a monounsaturated fat but is generally not recommended because most of the time it is genetically modified.

- Polyunsaturated fats include omega-3 fatty acids (fish oil) and omega-6 fatty acids (vegetable oil). Omega-3 fatty acids come mainly from fish such as wild Alaskan salmon, Alaskan black cod, and sardines. Other sources of omega-3 fats include walnuts, soybeans, and flaxseed. Omega-6 fatty acids include nuts, seeds, corn, soy, safflower, palm fruit, cottonseed, and canola. These fats are usually found in the diet in large amounts and are easy to obtain. They are good as long as they are not processed. Many processed foods such as cookies, crackers, sweets, and fast foods include refined vegetable oils, such as soy oil.

The Controversial Fat

Saturated fats are a type of single-bond animal or vegetable fat found in all meat and dairy products. Coconut and palm oil are also saturated fats. For many years, driven by commercial food corporations, the belief was that saturated fats should be limited since they were thought to increase blood cholesterol levels;

however, continuing research has revealed that saturated fats with medium and short chain fatty acids, such as those found in butter or coconut oil, are beneficial.[15]

Watch for continuing research on this controversial topic, which began back in the 1950s with some bad science that underplayed the role of sugar in causing heart disease and overrated the role of fats. The misconception that saturated fats and cholesterol raise blood cholesterol, which has been rampant in the past 30 years, was largely promoted by the food industry for their commercial gain.[16]

Really-Bad-for-You Fats

Trans fats, originally generated as a substitute for saturated fats, include hydrogenated and partially hydrogenated oils. These are commonly found in commercial cookies, crackers, margarine, and peanut butter. It turns out that trans fats are much worse for you than saturated fats and should be avoided.

The healthiest fat sources in general are: avocados, nuts (including walnuts, almonds, cashews, and peanuts), nut butters (natural peanut, almond, or cashew butters without added trans fats), olive oil, olives, ground flaxseed, and seeds (pumpkin, sesame, and sunflower).

Putting It All Together

How much of each macronutrient should you consume? If you have had your APO E gene test done as a part of an APO E gene program, you will receive a diet and exercise program developed specifically for your body composition and your genetic type. If you have not had your APO E genotype determined, Dr. Andrew Weil's anti-inflammatory food pyramid is an excellent guideline to follow for healthy nutrition.[17]

Dr. Weil recommends eating four to five vegetables per day, both raw and cooked, from all parts of the color spectrum. He advises eating organic fruits and vegetables when possible (more on this a bit later). He also recommends three to four fruit servings a day, again organic when possible. He suggests three to five whole grain servings daily and one to two beans or legumes (beans, peas, and lentils) per day.

It is very important to eat organic foods when possible. More and more information is being generated about the negative consequences of genetically modified organisms (GMOs). A genetically modified organism is an organism whose genetic material has been altered using genetic engineering techniques (biotechnology). This experimental technology merges DNA from different species, creating unstable combinations of plant, animal, bacterial, and viral genes that cannot occur in nature. Virtually all commercial GMOs are engineered to withstand direct applications of herbicides or to produce insecticides. The most popular herbicide, glyphosate (found in Roundup), which had been touted as safe for decades has now been shown to be carcinogenic, with ever-increasing amounts of it found in our foods as plant resistance to it is requiring that higher and higher doses be applied to crops.[18] Despite biotech industry promises, none of the GMO products currently on the market offer increased yield, drought tolerance, enhanced nutrition, or any other consumer benefit.[19]

Besides the increasing carcinogenic herbicide exposure, two components of GMOs seem to be causing the most problems: Bt toxin and bovine growth hormone. Bovine growth hormone is injected into cows to increase their production of milk. Human consumption of milk that has bovine growth hormone has been implicated as a potential risk of cancer. Bt toxin is found in corn and is a natural soil-produced bacteria toxin. It can be used by organic farmers. When insects take in the Bt toxin, it causes their stomachs to explode, killing the insects. Bt toxin is washed off and is biodegradable.

Genetic engineers, however, have taken Bt toxin, made it 1,000 times more concentrated than the spray and have engineered it so it can't be washed off or biodegraded. According to the biotech company Monsanto, Bt toxin is supposed to be destroyed in the human gastrointestinal tract. However, Canadian scientists showed that Bt toxin was found in 93 percent of pregnant women and in 80 percent of their fetuses.[20]

Since GMOs have been introduced into our food crops, the incidence of gastrointestinal disorders such as irritable bowel syndrome, Crohn's disease, leaky gut syndrome, autoimmune disorders (such as Hashimoto's thyroiditis), allergies, and infertility have all increased significantly. Thirty years ago, it was rare to witness a young couple having difficulty conceiving a child. Now one in six couples has infertility issues.

In my work, I have found that when patients eat organic foods and avoid GMO products, their symptoms such as gastrointestinal disorders, allergies, headaches, or Hashimoto's thyroiditis commonly disappear.

The nine most common GMO crops are corn, canola, soy, cottonseed, sugar beets, Hawaiian papaya, crooked neck squash, some zucchini, and alfalfa. The biggest offenders are corn, soy, canola, and sugar beets. Any product that has sugar listed as an ingredient is generally 50 percent cane sugar and 50 percent sugar from sugar beets. To avoid GMOs, always use organic sources of corn, canola, and soy. Additionally, use products with organic raw cane sugar instead of refined sugar. You can download a list of companies that use non-GMO products online.[21]

Even worse is the ubiquitous additive, high fructose corn syrup (HFCS), found in most processed foods. HFCS increases the risk of obesity, diabetes, hypertension, and cardiovascular disease.[22] The Institute for Responsible Technology lists over 170 items that are derived from corn. Consumers are used to avoiding the major ones, such as HFCS, dextrose, corn syrup, and corn syrup solids, but many of the corn-derived products are labeled to avoid affiliation with HFCS.[23] Would you ever think that xanthan gum, bleached flour, food starch, baking powder, or iodized salt has corn in it? Researcher Stephan Macko has determined through hair analysis that for most Americans, 50 percent of their carbon makeup comes from corn.[24]

Each year, the Environmental Working Group publishes a list of the Clean Fifteen and the Dirty Dozen foods.[25] The Clean Fifteen foods are grown in a manner that has a low incidence of pesticide use, so it is reasonable to purchase them conventionally grown. Foods that are grown conventionally will have a bar code number that begins with the number four. The Dirty Dozen foods, on the other hand, are grown in a manner that has a high degree of pesticide use. These foods should be purchased only when they are organically grown. The bar code for organic fruits and vegetables always begins with the number nine.

Dirty Dozen Foods	Clean Fifteen Foods
These foods have a high degree of pesticide exposure and should be consumed only if grown organically.	*These foods have a lower degree of pesticide exposure and can be consumed safely if conventionally grown.*
1. Strawberries	1. Avocados
2. Apples	2. Sweet corn*
3. Nectarines	3. Pineapples
4. Peaches	4. Cabbage
5. Celery	5. Sweet peas (frozen)
6. Grapes	6. Onions
7. Cherries	7. Asparagus
8. Spinach	8. Mangos

9. Tomatoes	9. Papayas*
10. Sweet bell peppers	10. Kiwi
11. Cherry tomatoes	11. Eggplant
12. Cucumbers	12. Honeydew melon
	13. Grapefruit
	14. Cantaloupe
	15. Cauliflower

* A small amount of sweet corn, papaya, and summer squash sold in the United States is produced from GE (genetically engineered) seeds. Buy organic varieties of these crops if you want to avoid GE produce.

©Environmental Working Group, EWG.org. Reproduced with permission.

Restful Sleep

Sleep is important to help our bodies restore and regenerate. Seven to eight hours is typically recommended. The more sleep you can get before midnight, the better. If you have trouble falling asleep, it could be a sign of adrenal fatigue. Cortisol is highest in the morning and then decreases through the day, typically being lowest in the evening so you can fall asleep easily.

Have you ever experienced a second wind after ten p.m. and then had difficulty falling asleep when you actually do go to bed? This could be a symptom of adrenal stress or adrenal fatigue. It's important to go to bed before you get that second wind, so your cortisol level can be reset. Some have no problem falling asleep but awaken between two and three a.m. and have difficulty going back to sleep. Common causes are excessive stress levels, adrenal fatigue, hormonal imbalances (common after menopause), and eating a heavy meal with excessive protein too late in the evening. Here are tips to help you get more restful sleep: [26]

1. Gradually reduce the amount of caffeine you drink during the day. You may want to stop all caffeine after lunch. Consider decaffeinated beverages.

2. Allow your body to reset its own regenerative rhythms so that you don't depend on stimulants to keep you going.

3. Clear emotional reactions such as irritation, worry, anxiety, judgments, and blame as you go through the day, as this might be keeping you awake at night. Write down anything that is left over at the end of the day in order to clear your mind and help you relax.

4. Before turning out the lights, write down something amusing that happened to you that day.

5. Follow the rhythms of nature. Maximize the amount of sleep you get before midnight.

6. Create consistent sleep rituals before going to bed that relax you for a nice night of sleep.

   • Stop all electronics (computers, cell phones, TV, etc.) at least two hours before bedtime.

   • Have a cup of chamomile tea an hour before bedtime.

   • Take a soothing bath to relax your body.

   • Rub on some lavender oil to enhance sleep.

   • Listen to soothing music before falling asleep.

   • Use prayer, meditation, or HeartMath® (described in the next section) to create gratitude for the day before retiring.

- Limit exposure to negative or upsetting stimuli before bedtime. You may want to avoid watching your local news station before going to bed.

- Create total darkness in your bedroom. The absence of light produces the hormone melatonin, which plays an important role in your mental and physical well-being and improves your sleep quality.

HeartMath® has even more tips on overcoming sleeplessness on their website.[27]

Exercise

We are all aware that exercise is beneficial. Recent research has shown that exercise may slow the aging process. Carl Cotman, PhD, a leading researcher for Alzheimer's disease, discovered that a protein known as the brain-derived neurotrophic factor (BDNF) protects the animal brain against aging and is increased with exercise. He is now researching whether BDNF can slow the progress of Alzheimer's disease. In his studies, he tested two groups of mice: one group sat in a cage all night; the other group had access to an exercise wheel at night. After a time, he tested their brain function. Consistently the animals that exercised could learn faster and better than those animals that didn't exercise.[28]

Next Dr. Cotman tested animals that had Alzheimer's disease. These animals' brain function also improved with exercise. He documented that exercise induces growth factors in the brain, increases new neurons in the circuits, builds synapses, improves vascular function, and enhances ability to learn. No drug can do all this. This may motivate and inspire you to make exercise a priority in your schedule. It's never too late and never too early to begin an exercise program. Use the FITT principle when you begin:[29]

- Frequency: Begin gradually and work up to exercising most days of the week (five to six days). Find a balance that will provide enough stress for the body to challenge your exercise capacity and muscle strength, yet also allow enough rest time for healing between exercise sessions.

- Intensity: The amount of effort required to do the exercise should be difficult enough to stretch the body's exercise capacity, but not to reach the point that it results in overtraining, injury, or burnout.

- Time: The amount of time spent exercising will vary, depending on intensity and type.

- Type: What type of exercise will you do? Vary your exercise to make it more enjoyable. Aerobic exercises such as walking, tennis, jogging, and swimming are great for the body. Stretching exercises help improve muscle tone. Strength training exercises such as yoga, Pilates, resistance bands, or weights are also beneficial for your muscles. Doing a variety of movements and exercises will use different muscle groups, increase your cardiovascular performance, and keep you inspired to continue your exercise program.

In summary, this is how you increase your physical energy vibration to stay above the line:

- Drink at least 64 ounces of water daily.

- Eat healthy portions of all three macronutrients.

- Use non-GMO products and consume only organic soy, corn, canola, and sugar.

- Avoid high fructose corn syrup and hydrogenated oils.

- Exercise four to six days per week.

- Sleep at least seven to eight hours per night.

These steps will do your body good and help you achieve your optimal physical health.

Raising Your Vibration of Optimal Psychological/Emotional Health

Staying above the line psychologically and emotionally is just as important as staying above the line physically. On average, we have 60,000 thoughts per day. About 60–75 percent of these thoughts are typically negative. This is what I refer to as your "self-talk." It's very important to become aware of your own self-talk. Are your thoughts commonly negative or positive? If they are negative, you might have to change your "stinking thinking."

Here is why your thoughts are so important. Thoughts originate in the frontal cortex. The hypothalamus is closely connected to the frontal cortex. The master gland—the pituitary is attached just below the hypothalamus. Many neuropeptides, neurotransmitters, and chemical messengers originate here. Literally, thoughts and attitudes generate biochemical events, which affect every cell in your body.

Remember what was stated earlier about the Law of Attraction? Whatever frequency you are vibrating, you will attract a similar frequency back to yourself. This is particularly apparent with thoughts. Whatever you put your attention on is what expands in your reality. If your focus is on what you lack or if you fear that you don't have enough of something (e.g., money), what do you think you will attract? Conversely if you focus on abundance, how much you have and how grateful you are to have what you do, the universe will respond by generating more abundance. Do you see the glass as half full or half empty? Teach yourself to focus on gratitude and appreciation. Each night write down five things for which you are most grateful. This is a great exercise for the entire family. Encouraging children at an early age to create positive patterns of gratitude and appreciation can benefit them throughout their lives.

Managing emotions positively contributes greatly toward your psychological and emotional health yet can be challenging at times. Relationships—whether in your family, work, or social circles—may be a source of stress as well as pleasure. But remember the words of the late Wayne Dyer, PhD, who reminded us that there is no such thing as stress—only people having stressful thoughts.[30]

Ten percent is what happens to you and 90 percent is the attitude and meaning that you bring to it. Events are going to happen. How you respond to them is what makes them stressful or not. You may find that when you change the way you look at things, the things you look at change.[31]

Learn to accept yourself and everything that happens to you as an opportunity for growth and learning. Fear and excitement are similar energetic vibrations. So, if you feel fearful, take a breath and tell yourself you choose excitement instead of fear. When something happens that you don't particularly like, learn to step back, breathe, and accept that it's an opportunity to grow. Trust the process. Look for the silver lining in the experience.

Let's look at emotions from another perspective. Each one of us has the need for what my good friend and teacher, Gertrude Brumleve, calls the four As—attention, affection, acceptance, and approval.[32] We are born with what she calls "emotional dyslexia"— we don't know what these emotions are, but we know we need them. We are hardwired to first get the four As from outside ourselves— from our parents and extended family. Having these core needs met at an early age allows us to incorporate them into our psyche. The massive, but poorly recognized disconnection of people in modern society, has been created through medicalized birth, being carted around in wheeled containers instead of human arms, left to sleep alone in cages, and left to "cry it out."

The resulting unmet early needs of children are largely a result of the barely seen disaster of the failed nuclear family experiment— trying to meet the needs of a newborn with only one or two adults. It has created generations of disconnected adults who then try to get their unmet needs through their spouse, children, or grandchildren. These aspects of the current norms have been labeled coercion parenting.[33]

This is contrasted with connection parenting, which meets children's early needs in order for them to reach emotional maturity.[34] Only then, when their formative years have fulfilled their need for the four As, can emotional maturity be achieved, and we can then meet our own emotional needs through healthy, co-creative, interdependent relationships with peers. Negative emotions such as jealousy, anger, or fear can be viewed as a stimulus indicating that one or more of the four As are not being met. For instance, if I feel jealous, this is a signal that I need to give myself more affection. If I am feeling sad or hurt, I need to give myself more attention. Thus, negative emotions actually have a positive benefit.

Another useful concept in managing emotions is becoming aware of the mirroring phenomenon that often leads to some ancient trauma from our childhood being triggered. Imagine a time when someone really upset you. What were you feeling? Can you remember back to the first time you felt this way? What were the circumstances? What was happening at that time? You may think that person over there just ticked you off, and that it's their fault you are feeling angry. If this person weren't so mean or rude, you wouldn't feel the way you do, but rarely does our emotional response entirely result from the present circumstance. Instead, most of the time, this intense reaction has little or nothing to do with that person and indicates there is a hurt or need inside you that needs to be healed. Something has triggered an aspect of your "shadow"—the parts of your unconscious that you'd rather not know about.[35] That upsetting person is simply mirroring that "hole in your soul" that needs to be healed. Usually this is related to hidden traumas and emotions from the past. Owning your shadow projections is key to healing these past traumas and unhelpful emotions and improving your psychological health.

One of the key skills in personal wellness is to learn to recognize when we are triggered and then to take back the shadow we have projected onto the mirror-person. In this way, we can repair many of ruptures that result from our triggered reactivity. Spouses and other close family members are the most exquisite source of personal mirrors. We often choose spouses because they have similar behavior patterns to those with whom we grew up.[36] Gaining the tools to help heal ourselves, ideally with the support of the other, is paramount to maintaining long-lasting, deep relationships.[37]

You may require professional help in order to identify, treat, and heal past wounds or traumas. It takes some work and emotional maturity to admit that we each are responsible for managing our emotions. It's much easier to blame the other person and ignore the fact that this could have anything to do with ourselves. Once you identify and begin to heal the source of a trigger, you may find that this person no longer emotionally stimulates you. I once heard this phenomenon described as "Name it, claim it, tame it." Once you identify and acknowledge the trigger, the emotional response lessens or disappears altogether. If you find that you are continuing to be emotionally triggered by a person or situation, the source of the underlying trauma or trigger may be so deeply subconscious that it will warrant professional help to bring these issues to your conscious awareness.

As we grow emotionally, we realize that we are each here to love and appreciate each other. And, the more we learn to love and appreciate ourselves, and all our experiences, good and bad, the more we can love and appreciate others.

Despite there being "no such thing as stress," it surely is pervasive in our society. Stress costs America more than $300 billion in lost productivity.[38] Of the 14 common symptoms responsible for half of all primary care visits, only 10–15 percent were found to have an organic cause.[39] At least 80 percent of the primary care visits are stress-induced or stress-related.[40] Managing stressful events and stressful feelings is an important part of staying above the line psychologically and emotionally.

Here are ways to manage your stressors:

- Breathing exercises are a wonderful way to help manage the physiological and psychological effects of stress. When you feel stressed, that fight-or-flight sensation in your body increases, due to the stimulation of your sympathetic nervous system. Your cortisol and adrenaline increase, causing your blood pressure, heart rate, and blood sugar to all increase as well. Simply taking some slow, deep breaths can calm the sympathetic response and allow the parasympathetic nervous system—the relaxed part of your nervous system—to be dominant. Remember Dr. Weil's 4-7-8 breathing technique that I described in chapter 5? This is a great way to calm your stressful response.

- The HeartMath® Institute describes the heart as the GPS of the body. It surprised me to learn that more messages go from my heart to my brain than from my brain to my heart. HeartMath® Institute has shown that when you focus on feelings of gratitude, appreciation, and love, your heart achieves a rhythmic coherence. When you are stressed and anxious, this heart rhythm is chaotic and incoherent. Try an experiment now: Get into a relaxed position. Take a few deep breaths. Now imagine your breath moving in and out through your heart. If it helps, put your hand on your heart. Think of a time when you felt gratitude and appreciation. Feel it as if it is happening right now. Breathe slowly in this space of love and gratitude for several minutes. How do you feel? Chances are you feel much more relaxed and happier and may even notice your thinking is a bit clearer. HeartMath® has done extensive research and offers solutions for stress.[41]

- Expand and enhance your sense of humor. Humor is a fabulous anecdote for stress. My colleague Clifford Kuhn, MD, known as the Laugh Doctor, has spent years researching the positive benefits of humor and has cleverly summarized this as the HaHaHa prescription.[42]

  - The first Ha stands for humor attitude. Many of us have trivialized humor and suppressed our humorous nature to be serious and "professional." Yet, our humorous nature can be a wonderful tool to increase the fun and enjoyment in our lives.

  - The second Ha stands for humor aptitude. As you begin to trust your humorous nature, you will find a natural inclination for humor and fun. I have found this to be true. The more I allow myself to laugh and enjoy life, the more funny things I notice. Isn't this a more fun way to go through your day?

○ The third Ha is humor action. As you appreciate the value of humor in your life and its ability to eradicate your stress, you will be inspired to act to enhance the presence of fun and laughter in your life. There are many ways to enhance your sense of humor: smile, read the comics, think of something that made you laugh, tell a humorous story to a friend, or hang out with funny people. When you subscribe to the HaHaHa prescription, you will be amazed at how much fun and enjoyment naturally expands in your life.

To summarize, this is how you raise your vibration, psychologically and emotionally, to stay above the line:

1. Change your stinking thinking.

2. Keep your self-talk positive.

3. Choose the feeling of excitement vs. fear.

4. Learn to manage your emotions.

5. Use some or all of the listed strategies to lower your stress level and increase your feelings of fun and enjoyment.

These strategies will help you create your optimal psychological and emotional health.

Raising Your Vibration for Optimal Spiritual Health
Last, but by no means least, is spiritual health, the most important. As I stated previously, we are spiritual beings having a human experience. Spirituality is the essence of who we truly are. Some have described

this spiritual essence as our soul or spirit. This essence transcends our body-mind complex, as I explained in the previous chapter.

Spirituality is not the same as religion. While some people may enhance their spirituality through organized religion, this is not the case for everyone. Spiritual essence is our connection to the Divine (God, Absolute, Higher Power, Source). (Please note: From here on I will refer to God as the Divine Essence or Source of all that is. Feel free to substitute your description within the context of your own beliefs.)

It's impossible to not be connected to the Divine. We are each a part of this Divine Essence. Imagine if the Divine were an ocean. Think of each of us as a single wave in that ocean. A wave could not be disconnected from the ocean—similarly, we can never be disconnected from the Divine.

The term spirituality is derived from the Latin word spiritus, meaning breath, referring to the vital spirit or soul.[43] Think of the word "inspiration." Literally when you inspire, you are "in spirit" and connected to spirit with each breath. Spirituality has been described as the way we find meaning, hope, comfort, and inner peace. Some may experience these aspects through religious practices, while others find spirituality through music, art, or a connection with nature.[44] Spirituality shapes, and is shaped by, our life journey. It is expressed and experienced through our connection with the Sacred Source, the self, others and/or nature.[45]

Since we are all part of Divine Essence, we are also all part of the body of humanity. Just like the 30 trillion or so cells that make up the physical body, we are each a unique part of the body of humanity. It would be absurd for the left hand to cut off the right hand, and equally absurd that one part of humanity would bomb or injure another part of it. We are all part of and connected to the same Divine Essence. Science is beginning to prove this innate divine connection. If you look at a cell under a microscope, you will find that the smallest components of the cell are not particles at all but are waves of energy. Further experiments have supported the fact that a web of energy connects us all. Consider the following experiment described by Gregg Braden.[46]

During the 1990s, scientists working in the US Army investigated whether the power of our feelings has an effect on DNA once it is removed from the body. Cheek swab samples from volunteers were taken to obtain their DNA. The cells containing the DNA were isolated, transported to another room down the hall and placed in a specially designed chamber so the DNA samples could be measured electrically. The volunteers were then shown films to evoke different emotions of fear, excitement, love, or humor. It was discovered that when the donors experienced emotional reactions, their cells and DNA showed powerful electrical responses at exactly the same time, despite being separated by hundreds of feet. This same experiment was repeated at greater distances, the farthest being 350 miles and the response continued to be similar and instantaneous.[47] How could this be?

These experiments support that there is an energy field that connects us all. This energy field is becoming recognized as the connection between science and spirituality. This energy field is everywhere. There is nowhere that the Divine is not. Gregg Braden concluded that this energy field and the Divine are synonymous. He refers to this energy field as the Divine Matrix.[48]

Knowing that everything is energy, even our thoughts, it's logical to see that our thoughts have an impact far beyond ourselves. Have you ever had the experience of thinking of someone and then shortly afterward you either see them or they call you? Acknowledging the existence of the Divine Matrix and that thoughts are energy that can travel through this matrix, it's easy to see how this can happen. It's not just a coincidence—it's science.

Our thoughts and energy are all contributing to this Divine Matrix or field of energy. Not only do we contribute to the Divine Matrix, but we can tap into this field at any time. Tapping into this matrix is our access to manifesting miracles. Access can be enhanced by our thoughts, prayer, or meditation. In his landmark book, *Healing Words: The Power of Prayer and the Practice of Medicine*, Larry Dossey proved that prayer made a difference toward the positive outcomes of patients, even without their awareness that prayers were being said for them.[49]

Prayer has been a mainstay in my life. In my most difficult times, prayer has provided comfort and allowed me to trust in the Divine—knowing that even though I can't see the whole picture from my human perspective, I can surrender to Divine guidance and allow the situation to unfold in divine perfection. This is not painless, yet trust in the Divine provides hope. The body's response to hope is an entirely different chemical reaction than the body's response to fear. Hope creates an anticipatory energy that waits to see how the Divine will unfold. Many times, it's been beyond what I could have imagined.

Consider my friend Amy. In the same week, she lost her nurse practitioner job, and her fiancé broke up with her. I told her that she had just experienced the "double cosmic kick," and I felt that something great was about to unfold for her. Of course, this was a difficult time for her emotionally. I sent her cards and had many conversations to inspire and encourage her. Despite her pain, she continued to trust the process and know that it was all in divine order. She remained hopeful, even though the recent events of her life were beyond her human understanding. Within six months, she met the man of her dreams and was offered another nurse practitioner position that she loved even more than her previous job.

Love is the language, the manifestation, of the Divine. Our main purpose is to love each other and support each other. It is through our relationships that this is most easily recognized and expressed. In the busyness of our day-to-day lives, it's easy to forget that our divine purpose is to love and support each other. Instead, we sometimes align with the vibrations of fear, anger, frustration, confusion, and guilt. You can easily see on the energy model that these low vibrational frequencies are away from the Divine. We always have free will and the choice to change our thoughts, change our feelings, and do something to raise our vibration above the line and back toward the Divine.

We are each unique expressions of the Divine. We are here to enjoy our human existence and co-create with the Divine. As we expand our conscious awareness, we begin to see that when we align our vibrational frequencies to those of love, happiness, kindness, generosity, and joy, i.e., the language and manifestation of the Divine, we find our true spiritual purpose.

We find that life truly is a co-creation and partnership with the Divine. We can consciously choose to align our thoughts and emotions with our spiritual essence to create the life we were meant to have, or we can choose to align with fear, confusion, frustration, and negativity. It's all energy. Whatever vibration we create is the frequency we will attract. Now you can appreciate the importance of aligning with the vibrations of love, gratitude, happiness, and joy.

How do we know we are in alignment with our spiritual essence? First, pay attention to how you feel. Are you naturally happy? Are you at peace? Are you content with how your life is going? These are indicators of divine alignment. Secondly, watch for divine synchronicities—those little, seeming coincidences that are inexplicable—signs from the Divine that you are in alignment. These synchronicities are divine miracles. Sometimes they are small and sometimes they are life changing.

For instance, in my practice, it is quite common that, if a patient calls to reschedule an appointment due to an unforeseen circumstance, another patient will call and ask if there is any opening. I refer to these synchronistic moments as "the angels doing the schedule." Perfect divine miracles.

Some of the divine synchronicities have literally been life changing. In 2003, I set the intention to write this book. I told my husband that I needed to attend a publishing class and that I wanted to visit the North Waimea Hospital on the Big Island of Hawai'i. One week after I said that, I received a flyer from the National Nurses in Business Association advertising an upcoming seminar that included a four-hour publishing segment. Three weeks later, I received a brochure from the American College of Cardiology. They were co-sponsoring an integrative medicine and cardiology program with the North Waimea Hospital!

I knew I was meant to attend both of these conferences. In Hawai'i, I met my colleague Pam McDonald, who is also an integrative medicine nurse practitioner. She had recently begun her own practice as well. That divine meeting was the start of a friendship and colleagueship that literally changed and expanded the trajectory of my life far beyond what I could have imagined.

Life is not always easy. As spiritual beings having a human experience, we are meant to experience all human emotions. This may include pain, suffering, love, happiness, and forgiveness (especially for ourselves). It's important that, even though we may not always understand the grand divine plan, we accept all that is, trust the process, and remain consciously connected to the Divine.

I have learned not to over-react if something is not happening as I planned, or an event is not going the way I thought it would. Commonly I find that, with time, and a bit of patience, divine perfection is revealed, and I realize the events were all in divine order. One of my favorite quotes is excerpted from Max Ehrmann's poem, "Desiderata": "And whether or not it is clear to you, no doubt the Universe is unfolding as it should."[50]

In summary, this is how you can raise your spiritual vibration and achieve optimal spiritual health to stay above the line:

- Consciously connect to Divine Essence (God, Source, Absolute) every day through prayer, meditation, or spending time in nature.

- Love daily (especially yourself).

- Appreciate all that life has to offer.

- Trust the divine plan—know that the universe always has your back.

- Watch for divine synchronicities as proof that God is present.

When you put it all together and raise your vibration physically, psychologically, emotionally, and spiritually, you will create your optimal health of mind, body, and spirit.

---

1. Mayo Clinic, "Dementia," Mayo Clinic website, https://www.mayoclinic.org/diseases-conditions/dementia/symptoms-causes/syc-20352013, accessed October 23, 2017.

2. Institute of Medicine, "Dietary Reference Intakes: Electrolytes and Water," National Agricultural Library, United States Department of Agriculture website, https://www.nal.usda.gov/sites/default/files/fnic_uploads//electrolytes_water.pdf, accessed October 23, 2017.

3. Janet Mentes, "Oral Hydration in Older Adults: Greater Awareness is Needed in Preventing, Recognizing, and Treating Dehydration," *American Journal of Nursing* 106, no. 6 (2006): 40–49.

4. Ibid.

5. McDonald, *Perfect Gene Diet.*

6. Institute for Integrative Medicine, (502) 253-4554 or integrativemedicine4u.com; Pam McDonald, Penscott Medical, (925) 736-8510 or https://apoegenediet.com/.

7. Self-Nutrition Data, "Glycemic Index," Self-Nutrition Data website, http://nutritiondata.self.com/topics/glycemic-index, accessed October 23, 2017.

8. Centers for Disease Control and Prevention, "Key Elements of Healthy Eating Patterns" in *Dietary Guidelines, 2015–2020*, CDC website, https://health.gov/dietaryguidelines/2015/guidelines/chapter-1/a-closer-look-inside-healthy-eating-patterns/#callout-dietary-fats, accessed October 23, 2017.

9. Tracey Roizman, "Do Hormones in the Food Supply Affect the Human Body?" *SF GATE*, https://healthyeating.sfgate.com/hormones-food-supply-affect-human-body-2194.html, accessed October 23, 2017.

10. Samuel S. Epstein, "Hormones in US Beef Linked to Increased Cancer Risk," October 21, 2009, Organic Consumers Association website, https://www.organicconsumers.org/news/hormones-us-beef-linked-increased-cancer-risk.

11. *Food, Inc.*, Robin Schorr, Jeff Skoll, and Diane Weyermann, executive producers; Robert Kenner, director and producer, Magnolia Pictures, 2008, documentary film.

12. Vital Choice website, https://www.vitalchoice.com/, accessed October 23, 2017.

13. *Forks over Knives*, Brian Wendel, executive producer and Lee Fulkerson, director, Monica Beach Media, 2011, documentary film.

14. *Forks over Knives* documentary film; and Gene Stone, ed. *Forks over Knives: The Plant-Based Way to Health* (New York: The Experiment, 2011).

15. Joseph Mercola, *Fat for Fuel: A Revolutionary Diet to Combat Cancer, Boost Brain Power, and Increase Your Energy* (Carlsbad, CA: Hay House, 2017).

16. Andreas Eenfeldt, "The Hidden Truth Behind Ancel Keys' Famous Fat Graph," September 19, 2016, Diet Doctor website, https://www.dietdoctor.com/the-hidden-truth-behind-ancel-keys-famous-fat-graph.

17. Andrew Weil, "Dr. Weil's Anti-Inflammatory Food Pyramid," Dr. Weil's website, https://www.drweil.com/diet-nutrition/anti-inflammatory-diet-pyramid/dr-weils-anti-inflammatory-food-pyramid/, accessed October 23, 2017.

18. Environmental Protection Agency, Office of Pesticide Programs, "Glyphosate Issue Paper: Evaluation of Carcinogenic Potential," September 12, 2016, EPA website, https://www.epa.gov/sites/production/files/2016-09/documents/glyphosate_issue_paper_evaluation_of_carcincogenic_potential.pdf; and Jeffrey M. Smith, "GMO FAQs," Institute for Responsible Technology website, http://responsibletechnology.org/gmo-education/faqs/, accessed October 23, 2017.

19. EPA, "Glyphosate Issue Paper"; and Jeffrey M. Smith, *Seeds of Deception. Exposing Industry and Government Lies About the Safety of the Genetically Engineered Foods You're Eating* (Fairfield, IA: Yes! Books, 2002).

20. Jeffrey M. Smith, "Are Genetically Modified Foods a Gut-Wrenching Combination?" Institute for Responsible Technology website, http://responsibletechnology.org/glutenintroduction/, accessed October 23, 2017.

21. Non-GMO Shopping Guide website, https://www.nongmoshoppingguide.com/, accessed October 23, 2017.

22. Dana Flavin, "Metabolic Dangers of High-Fructose Corn Syrup," *Life Extension* magazine website, http://www.lifeextension.com/magazine/2008/12/Metabolic-Dangers-of-High-Fructose-Corn-Syrup/Page-01, accessed October 23, 2017.

23. "Corn Products and Derivatives List," Institute for Responsible Technology website, https://responsibletechnology.org/irtnew/wp-content/uploads/2017/06/Corn-Products-Derivatives-06-06-17.pdf, accessed October 23, 2017.

24. "Corn, Corn, Everywhere Corn," Institute for Responsible Technology website, https://responsibletechnology.org/corn-corn-everywhere-corn/, accessed October 23, 2017.

25. "Shopper's Guide to Pesticides in Produce: Clean Fifteen and Dirty Dozen Foods," Environmental Working Group website, https://www.ewg.org/foodnews/, accessed October 23, 2017.

26. HeartMath® Institute, "Top Tips for Better Sleep," HeartMath® Institute website, https://www.HeartMath®.com/articles/top-tips-for-better-sleep/, accessed October 23, 2017.

27. Deborah Rozman and Rollin McCraty, *HeartMath® Solution for Better Sleep: Resetting Your Body's Rhythms, Integrating emWave and Inner Balance Technologies* (Boulder Creek, CA: HeartMath® LLC, 2013).

28. Carl Cotman, "Diet and Exercise in Alzheimer's," part of *The Alzheimer's Project,* a presentation of HBO Documentary Films and the National Institute on Aging at the National Institutes of Health, 2009.

29. Brad Walker, "The FITT Principle: Frequency, Intensity, Time, Type and How They Relate to Injury," Stretch Coach website, http://stretchcoach.com/articles/fitt-principle/, first published September 24, 2003; updated May 23, 2017; accessed October 23, 2017.

30. Wayne Dyer, *The Power of Intention: Learning to Co-Create Your World Your Way* (Carlsbad, CA: Hay House, 2010).

31. Ibid.

32. Gertrude Brumleve, "Emotional Maturity: What Is It?" Presentation at Institute for Integrative Medicine, Louisville, KY, September 27, 2002.

33. "Proclamation for Transforming the Lives of Children," Alliance for Transforming the Lives of Children website, http://atlc.org/Proclamation/proclamation.php, accessed October 23, 2017.

34. Pam Leo, *Connection Parenting: Parenting through Connection Instead of Coercion, through Love Instead of Fear,* 2nd ed. (Deadwood, OR: Wyatt-MacKenzie, 2007).

35. Robert Bly, *A Little Book on the Human Shadow* (San Francisco: HarperOne, 1988).

36. Alain de Botton, "Why You Will Marry the Wrong Person," *New York Times* website, https://www.nytimes.com/2016/05/29/opinion/sunday/why-you-will-marry-the-wrong-person.html, accessed October 23, 2017.

37. Susan Campbell and John Grey, *Five-Minute Relationship Repair: Quickly Heal Upsets, Deepen Intimacy, and Use Differences to Strengthen Love* (Novato, CA: New World Library, 2015).

38. "Workplace Stress," American Institute of Stress website, https://www.stress.org/workplace-stress/, accessed October 23, 2017.

39. Wayne Katon and Ed Walker, "Medically Unexplained Symptoms in Primary Care," *Journal of Clinical Psychology*, 59, supplement 20 (1998): 15–21.

40. A. Perkins, "Saving Money by Reducing Stress," *Harvard Business Review* 72, no. 6 (1994): 12.

41. HeartMath® Institute, "Solutions for Stress," HeartMath® Institute website, https://www.HeartMath®.org/resources/solutions-for-stress/reducing-stress/, accessed October 23, 2017.

42. Clifford Kuhn, *It All Starts with a Smile* (Louisville, KY: Butler Books, 2007).

43. Margaret A. Burkhardt and Mary Gail Nagai-Jacobson, "Spirituality and Health" in *Holistic Nursing: A Handbook for Practice*, 6th ed., eds. Barbara Montgomery Dossey and Lynn Keegan (Burlington, NH: Jones & Bartlett, 2013).

44. Gowri Anandarajah and Ellen Hight, "Spirituality and Medical Practice: Using the HOPE Questions as a Practical Tool for Spiritual Assessment," *American Family Physician* 63, no. 1 (2001): 81–89.

45. Anandarajah and Hight, "Spirituality and Medical Practice."

46. Braden, *Divine Matrix.*

47. J. Motz, "Everyone an Energy Healer: The Treat V Conference, Santa Fe, NM," *The Journal of Mind-Body Health* 9 (1993).

48. Braden, *Divine Matrix*

49. Larry Dossey, *Healing Words: The Power of Prayer and the Practice of Medicine* (New York: Harper Collins, 1993).

50. Max Ehrmann, "Desiderata," All Poetry website, https://allpoetry.com Desiderata—Words-for-Life, originally published 1927.

CHAPTER 8

A New Paradigm for Elder Care

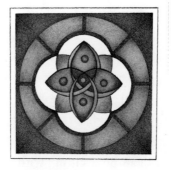

Have you noticed how Americans today are aging differently than their parents and grandparents? Many are remaining active and youthful long after the age that their parents ceased being healthy and youthful. One of my favorite patients is 90 years young. She first came to see me about five years ago because she noticed that without her estrogen cream, she was developing more facial wrinkles. She also wanted to try natural formulas and modalities for her increasing blood pressure since she had not tolerated any of the anti-hypertensive medications her primary care provider had prescribed. She looks at least 20 years younger than her actual age. She lives alone and manages her own household. She is active with her church, sings in the choir, and attends every University of Louisville men's home basketball game. She truly is my idol.

One of my patients has a summer home at the Villages in Central Florida. This community is for people aged 55 and older. They have 39 nine-hole golf courses and the main mode of transportation within the Villages is a golf cart. This community is one of the most active retirement communities that I've seen. They even sponsor senior games every March in which residents can compete in pickleball, tennis, swimming, running, polo games, and more. There is something for everyone. This is the new paradigm for healthy aging.

Have you heard the familiar adage, "The only constant in life is change?" This is certainly true with aging, as it is inevitable that our lives and circumstances will change. Most of us will retire from our work obligations and perhaps have more free time. This might give us additional time to travel, spend time with our spouse, children, grandchildren, friends, and neighbors. We might choose to increase our involvement in church activities, volunteer work, or social causes. This phase of our lives can be exciting, with new opportunities to grow, learn, and experience.

As we baby boomers enter our elder years, we are not going to settle for the kind of elder care that our parents and grandparents might have received in nursing homes or long-term care facilities. Evidence of this is readily identifiable. Every city is creating new retirement facilities that focus on providing active lifestyles for residents. Many offer daily exercise classes such as Tai Chi, Pilates, water aerobics, swimming, or yoga. Many of these facilities also sponsor activities to encourage socialization and the opportunity to develop new friendships.

Traditional nursing homes are being recreated and redesigned. Consider what Bill Thomas, MD, did as medical director of Chase Memorial Nursing Home, in New Berlin, New York, in 1991.[1] As a new medical director, he identified the three plagues of nursing home existence:

- Boredom

- Loneliness

- Helplessness

He had a radical idea of bringing life into the nursing home. He proposed to management that they apply for a small New York State grant that was available for innovative programs for the elderly.

The administrator agreed to apply for the grant, which included putting live green plants in every room and creating a vegetable and flower garden on the lawn. The application also included funds to acquire and care for four cats, two dogs and a hundred parakeets. The administrator went along with this seemingly preposterous proposal, never expecting that the grant would be approved, but to his dismay, not only was the grant approved, but all the necessary waivers were given to allow the animals into the nursing home.

The results were literally amazing. Staff members brought their children to hang out after school. Friends and family built a garden at the back of the home and a playground for the children. The effect on the residents was miraculous. Elders who had previously not talked began to speak. One elderly gentleman, who had been completely withdrawn and non-ambulatory, approached the nursing staff and offered to walk the dog. All 100 birds were adopted and named by residents. Even more astounding was that the number of prescription medications required per resident fell to half that of a control group nursing home over the next two years.

Since then, Dr. Thomas, who describes himself as the "Ambassador of Elderhood," has created a nonprofit organization called the Eden Alternative, whose mission is "to improve the well-being of elders and their care partners by transforming the communities in which they live and work."[2] The Eden Alternative emphasizes 10 principles to combat the three plagues of the elderly—loneliness, boredom, and helplessness.

The Eden Alternative principles are:

1. Create a cultural shift from institutional models of care to person-directed values and practices, which put the elders first.

2. Commitment to creating a human habitat of abounding life with plants, animals, and children.

3. Acknowledge that loving companionship is the antidote to loneliness.

4. Create opportunities to give care as well as receive care. This focus pairs elder storytellers with recording partners who are at least 16 years old and who record the elder's story and legacy.

5. Imbue life with variety and spontaneity to allow unexpected and unpredictable interactions to happen. This is the antidote to boredom.

6. Opportunities are created for elders to do things that are meaningful. This is viewed as essential to human health.

7. Medical treatment is viewed as the servant of genuine human caring and never its master.

8. Honor elders by de-emphasizing top-down bureaucratic authority. Seek instead to place the maximum possible decision-making authority into the hands of the elders or those closest to them.

9. Elder-centered communities are a never-ending process. Human growth must never be separated from human life.

10. Wise leadership is the lifeblood of any struggle against the three plagues. For it, there is no substitute.[3]

Dr. Thomas reminds us that we are all elders in the making. He is on a mission to radically change the culture of aging worldwide. In 2016, Dr. Thomas traveled all around the country presenting his Age of Disruption bus tour, which challenges our national obsession with remaining young, and advocates the beauty and value of elderhood. Dr. Thomas states, "Aging is the least understood part of the human life span and, potentially, the richest and most meaningful. Aging is an active, growth-oriented process and not a passive, decline-oriented process."[4] Not only have we as a society ignored the value of aging, we have even tried to prevent it with anti-aging medicine.

Dr. Thomas has been instrumental in creating and supporting the Green House Project, which is a movement to transform traditional long-term care away from an institutional model and into small community-based homes. At this writing, there are 187 Green House residences in 13 states across America.

Each Green House cottage houses 12 residents, who have their own bedroom and bathroom. All the other areas of the home are shared, including the kitchen, living room with hearth, den, and porch area. Elders can grow and thrive with other residents while receiving any needed individualized care. Outcomes have been extraordinary for both residents and the staff. The residents feel as if they are at home and not in an institution. Their quality of life and emotional health are improved. They feel loved, acknowledged, and well cared for. There are fewer resident falls, fewer hospitalizations, and a decreased use of psychotropic medications compared to conventional long-term care facilities. The staff is completely empowered to create a home environment focused on the residents. This results in increased job satisfaction and significantly lower staff turnover. In this loving environment, morale is high for residents and staff.

In Kentucky, the Homeplace at Midway is a Green House Residence. It is built in the Bluegrass Region on beautiful grounds next to Midway College, so that residents may enjoy lifelong learning. Also planned are garden homes for those who continue to live independently. What an inviting senior living community.

What if this reverence for elders continued into end-of-life care? It's well documented that most healthcare expenditures occur in the last two weeks to two months of a person's life.[5] This is very apparent in the intensive care unit (ICU) where we have expensive care and technology. In many instances, intensive care is lifesaving. At the same time, the average mortality rate for patients in ICUs across the nation is 10–19 percent.

There is an underlying attitude present in medicine and many hospital cultures that the death of a patient is some kind of failure on the part of the medical system. When a patient dies, there's often an undertone of failure, which can drive interventions and treatments beyond what is reasonable care for expected outcomes. These situations present complex emotional issues. As such, many factors of care become based on fears and legalistic strategies instead of reasonable achievable outcomes for patients.

For instance, if patients realized that only 8 percent of those who have a cardiac arrest in hospital settings regain their pre-arrest condition, they might decline to have full resuscitative measures executed.[6] Much of the over-care that happens in ICUs could be avoided with family education and communication. I commonly witnessed in the ICUs the providing of care long after a reasonable possible outcome could be realized.

Even when efforts were futile, aggressive care still would be given. Sometimes this was because family members could not agree on what reasonable care looked like or what their loved one would have wanted. Sometimes care was continued for legalistic priorities (i.e., fear of a lawsuit if every possible intervention was not attempted). I often felt that if patients could speak for themselves, they might have charged us with assault and battery for continuing their care beyond reasonable achievable goals. It was that futile!

Living Wills, Durable Powers of Attorney, and Advance Directives

Living wills can be very helpful for family members of patients who become too ill to participate in decisions regarding their end-of-life care. A living will might include preferences regarding blood transfusions, cardiopulmonary resuscitation, dialysis, and use of a ventilator if the individual becomes too ill to speak. It might also be beneficial to designate a durable power of attorney, not only for financial matters, but also for healthcare. This person oversees the patient's care if she or he becomes too ill to make healthcare decisions. Many states combine a living will and durable power of attorney into one legal document called an advance directive. These documents are separate from a traditional will executed after one dies. In Kentucky, one legal document, the advance directive, can suffice for the living will and durable power of attorney. Be sure to check your own state guidelines when creating your advance directive.

As healthcare providers, we must acknowledge that death is a natural part of the life process. Yes, life process. We were all born, and we are going to die. We need to shift our current belief and attitudes regarding death as failure and acknowledge that it's a natural part of a life cycle. Viewing death as a normal part of life may help us to be more emotionally adept at helping patients and families deal with end-of-life issues. Our goal is to provide optimal healthcare on the entire spectrum from birth through the death process.

End-of-life care can be highly emotional and variable, and it must be based on the needs of each individual. As care providers, we must continue to improve our communication skills and sensitivity to patients and families who are grieving. They may be confronting mortality issues, spiritual beliefs, or experiencing any of Dr. Elisabeth Kübler Ross's five stages of grief (denial, anger, bargaining, depression, and acceptance).[7]

Imagine if we had stronger support for families to deal with grief and death. Imagine if hospitals had a bereavement team. Many hospitals use chaplains in these roles. Some hospitals have created palliative care units that are designed to provide end-of-life care, based on comfort and compassion versus extraordinary, oftentimes futile, treatments.

One area of grief that is commonly overlooked in hospital settings is support for the healthcare staff. In my work as the critical care specialist, I witnessed deaths that were anticipated and expected. Yet occasionally unexpected deaths occurred and came as a total shock. These times were difficult, not only for the families, but also for the staff. In such situations, nurses and physicians caring for these patients had to suppress their own emotions of sadness, grief, or guilt, process them quickly, and go right on to meet the next patient's needs without missing a beat.

Over time, this is not a healthy pattern. Suppressing or ignoring these feelings can lead to compartmentalization, callousness, denial, and detachment from emotions. None of these are desirable characteristics for healthcare providers. Support mechanisms must be in place to help nurses, physicians, and other care providers to process and deal with their emotions.

What if things were different? What if caring for the patient and family included caring *through* the death process? What if families and healthcare providers were supported so that time and space could be given for all to acknowledge their grief? Imagine how beneficial it could be to families and care providers to include a component of care to honor and celebrate the patient's life when he or she died, regardless of how sudden, unexpected, or anticipated. Families could be encouraged to share with care providers aspects of their loved one's heroic journeys such as:

- What kind of person their loved one was

- What legacy their loved one left behind

- What their loved one stood for—their goals, aspirations, dreams, and achievements in life

Imagine a transition team of two or three providers who would come to a unit when a patient dies to support the dying patient's family and attending staff. This team could help console the family and the staff, or step in and care for the staff's other patients while their colleagues devoted time to the grieving family.

Planting the seed for a family to honor and celebrate their loved one's life could greatly help ease their emotional pain and grieving process. A celebration of a loved one's life might evoke a feeling of gratitude for the time that their family did have together. This could be a time for families to review the meaning and purpose of their loved one's life and honor their spirit as they transition to the next phase. This acknowledgement and celebration could even continue beyond the healthcare setting. Wouldn't that be a much healthier way to deal with death than how it's commonly done now?

While our human experience is temporary, our spiritual essence is eternal. If we all claimed this beyond a shadow of a doubt and knew that we will return to our Source of Oneness (All-ness, the Divine), imagine how different the world would be. There no longer would be a need for wars in the name of the Creator. We would treat each other with respect, knowing that we're all connected and part of the Divine Essence and wholeness. We would help each other, serve each other, and love each other. All experiences might be viewed as part of the divine process, with a knowing and trust that all events are in divine order. Viewing painful situations and circumstances through these lenses might help ease our hurts. Though we may not be able to understand certain painful and horrible situations from a human perspective, we could trust that there is an overall divine purpose.

If we all shared this perspective, death care could be transformed. No longer would healthcare providers feel as if they have somehow failed a person or family when someone dies. Death is a natural consequence of life. This does not mean that we will not be sad or hurt if and when our loved ones or patients die and make their transition. Of course, we will experience sorrow and pain. We will miss them. These feelings are a testimony to the love we share for our family members and patients. At the same time, if we are confident that all souls, that part of us that is eternal, will meet again on the other side, our human hurting might be eased.

I witnessed a beautiful example of this with my friend Millie. She is a holistic nurse who has had to witness two husbands and her son make their transition. When her son died at the age of 33, from ALS—amyotrophic lateral sclerosis, I attended the visitation at the funeral home and was surprised to see Millie in a bright yellow suit. The casket was closed and there were beautiful pictures all around the room of her son in happy, smiling moments up until two weeks before his death, when his baby daughter was born. One couldn't help but feel a stark difference from most funeral home visits. Of course, everyone was sad and hurting. But amidst the tears were laughter and an honoring of his entire life.

The next day I attended the funeral, and again I was amazed. His wife, daughter, and brother were all dressed in the traditional black. Then here came Millie with a white suit that had large purple and green flowers on it. Again, I had the distinct impression that Millie wanted to celebrate and honor her son's life despite her grief and sadness.

As baby boomers enter their elder years, many more people and families are going to be faced with end-of-life issues, simply due to the sheer numbers of boomers. Not only is this a pressing health issue, it's also going to force many of us to confront death and mortality issues.

The US Department of Health and Human Services Administration on Aging reported in 2012 that the population of people 65 and older has increased from 35 million in 2000 to 41.4 million in 2011 (an 18 percent increase), and the number is projected to increase to 79.7 million in 2040.[8] Ninety-five percent of people, when asked, say they want to die at home but currently 75 percent die in a hospital or long-term care facility.[9]

Tarron Estes is the founder of the Conscious Dying Institute, which is responding to people's desire for a loving, more natural death. Her transformative programs help people prepare for death, both personally and professionally, so they can "be authentically present as they encounter death in themselves, their families and friends."[10] She has created certificate programs for caregivers in order for them to "companion people through death as a rite of passage versus a medical event."[11] One of the certificate programs trains caregivers to be death doulas. Just as doulas help with the birthing process, doulas trained through the Conscious Dying Institute help people and their families with the sacred process of dying. What a beautiful concept!

The institute's mission is to "restore death and dying to its natural place in the sacred circle of life by creating a new wisdom-based culture of healing caregivers and professionals, practicing across all healthcare settings, who elevate the experience of end-of-life care."[12] Estes teaches practitioners to be open to the sacredness of death, to acknowledge the unexplainable, and to witness the transformative healing power of death.

I hope this chapter has helped to transform your view of elderhood. It is a privilege to reach this milestone. Our elders have much wisdom, courage, and experience to share. We must honor them by listening to their stories, calming their fears, and loving them for who they are and all they have done in their lives. Finally, when the time comes for the end of their human lives, let us help them transition in grace, peace, and dignity, acknowledging the sacredness of their divine passing. May we surround them with love and appreciation for all they have been in our lives and celebrate their human existence as part of our grief process.

My son and daughter both live in Hawai'i, so I usually visit them annually. On my trips, I have noticed the profound respect for the elderly intrinsic in the Hawaiian culture. Even strangers hold doors open for older people and readily assist them in any way possible. Most elderly are referred to as "Auntie" or "Uncle," whether they are a blood relative or not. This term of endearment projects love, tenderness, and great respect for the Hawaiian elders. Not only does this make the elderly feel appreciated and loved, it enriches younger generations by teaching them to respect their elders. Let us take heed and carry this practice into all of America.

---

1. Atul Gawande, *Being Mortal: Medicine and What Matters in the End* (New York: Picador, 2017).

2. "Mission, Vision, Values, Principles," Eden Alternative website, http://www.edenalt.org/about-the-eden-alternative/mission-vision-values/, accessed October 23, 2017.

3. Ibid.

4. Ibid.

5. Tom Ahrens, Valerie Yancey, and Marin Kollef, "Improving Family Communications at the End of Life: Implications for Length of Stay in the Intensive Care Unit and Resource Use," *American Journal of Critical Care* 12, no. 4 (July 2003).

6. Ibid.

7. Elisabeth Kübler Ross and Ira Byock, *On Death and Dying: What the Dying Have to Teach Doctors, Nurses, Clergy and Their Own Families* (New York: Scribner, 2011).

8. Administration on Aging, Administration for Community Living, and US Department of Health and Human Services, "A Profile of Older Americans: 2012."

9. Tarron Estes, Conscious Dying Institute website, http://www.consciousdyinginstitute.com/, accessed October 23, 2017.

10. Ibid.

11. Ibid.

12. Ibid.

CHAPTER 9

How Do We Make Healthcare Affordable?

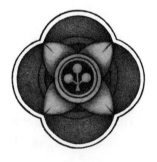

Our current disease-care system simply cannot be sustained economically. In *Why Our Health Matters*, Dr. Andrew Weil reports that the cost of American healthcare has increased from $8 billion in 1950 to $4 trillion in 2015.[1] This is an increase of 274 times what it was in 1950 when other industries, goods, and services have increased only an average of eight times. In the next seven to nine years, Dr. Weil projects that the cost of healthcare will probably go up 500 times what it was in 1950, even though the inflation rate over the next seven to nine years may be negligible. This is a wildfire out of control.

The amount we are spending on healthcare is consuming more and more of our annual gross domestic product (GDP). In 1960, healthcare spending comprised about 5 percent of our GDP. Current projections estimate that healthcare spending is expected to increase from 17.8 percent of the GDP in 2015 to 19.9 percent by 2025.[2]

In 1996, the money spent on Medicare and Medicaid totaled 1 percent of total government spending. Today that figure is over 20 percent and rising. If the future spending predictions are accurate, within 10 years, we could be spending 33 percent of the GDP (one third of the entire American economy) on Medicare and Medicaid.[3] Funding for all other public priorities such as education, environment, and public safety are dwindling because of this healthcare beast.[4] Continued escalation of healthcare costs will ruin the American economy. Already one in five Americans has so much medical debt that they are forced to pay through credit plans over time.[5] Medical debt is becoming the most common reason that Americans are filing for bankruptcy.

It would seem logical that if we are paying so much for healthcare, we must have one of the best healthcare systems in the world. Yet we rank 37th in healthiness compared to other industrialized nations.

Why is it that we spend so much on healthcare, yet our outcomes are not as good as many other countries around the world? Do you know of any other industry that would be able to remain in business with high costs and poor quality? Why do we as Americans allow this trend to exist and worse yet, continue? It's time for us to wake up and smell the roses. It's time for radical change in our healthcare system and its financing.

David Goldhill is a businessman who learned firsthand the perils of poor quality in healthcare. In 2007, his 83-year-old father, who was still working, developed pneumonia and was admitted to the local hospital. Within 36 hours, his condition deteriorated, and he was diagnosed with sepsis. He was moved to the intensive care unit where he developed a series of infections over the next five weeks that were largely determined to be hospital-acquired. Throughout these five weeks, Goldhill became intimately aware of the problems with the current healthcare system. He observed an infrastructure fraught with mistakes and the potential for errors. His father died, and as Goldhill describes in *The Atlantic*, he "became a statistic— merely one of the roughly 100,000 Americans whose deaths are caused or influenced by infections picked up in hospitals."[6]

Goldhill's experience with his father's hospitalization created in him a burning desire to look at this beast called healthcare. His knowledge and experience as a businessman afforded him the ability to draw some powerful conclusions. First, our healthcare models are plagued with reverse economic incentives. Hospitals and providers bill for more services, and therefore are reimbursed more money when patients are sick or have complications. Following this logic, you can see that in the economic structure of healthcare, more money is realized when people are sick. The greater the number of sick people, the greater the potential to bill for services. Goldhill describes this in his book, *Catastrophic Care: Why Everything We Think We Know about Healthcare Is Wrong*, as one part of a "moral hazard."[7]

As consumers, we are often unaware of healthcare costs, since we are not directly paying for services ourselves. Instead we have intermediaries paying our healthcare costs: health insurance companies, Medicare, and Medicaid. Goldhill describes these intermediaries as "surrogates." Using surrogates in the payer process creates a huge disconnect for American consumers and provides the illusion that someone else is paying the bills for our healthcare. This is yet another facet of Goldhill's moral hazard. We are inclined to use more services since we have insurance and "someone else is paying for it." This is just what health insurance companies want: for us to expand and expand our use of services. Expanded services mean more revenue for them and their stockholders. But what is not appreciated is what this surrogate system really costs us, and who actually reaps the real benefits.

Let's look at profits in the healthcare market, which are staggering.

Here are the gross profits recorded for the end of 2016 for each of the major health insurers.

- UnitedHealth Group $13.3 billion[8]

- Anthem (Blue Cross/Blue Shield) $2.47 billion[9]

- Cigna $15.18 billion[10]

- Aetna $2.4 billion[11]

- Humana $9.37 billion[12]

Here are the annual compensations for their CEOs:[13]

- Stephen Hemsley, United Healthcare Group: In 2016, his compensation was estimated at $31.3 million. This represented a 55.8 percent increase compared to 2015 (which was $14.5 million due to exercising stock options.)[14]

- Joseph Swedish, Anthem $16.5 million

- David Cordani, Cigna $15.3 million

- Mark Bertolini , Aetna, $18.7 million

- Bruce Broussard, Humana $19.7 million

Even during the years from 2008 to 2010, when the country experienced a significant recession and most other industries were scaling back and laying off employees, healthcare expanded by adding 732,000 new jobs.[15] It seems that even during a financial crisis, healthcare costs continue to expand.

We have equated healthcare with health insurance. I believe this is quite apparent with the Affordable Care Act. This bill has done nothing to change the current infrastructure of the disease-care model. Instead we've just ensured that:

- Everyone will participate in this dysfunctional system.

- "Healthcare" will continue to grow.

- More of us will continue to feed the profit margins of third-party insurers.

- Healthcare will continue to consume a higher percentage of our GDP.

Goldhill describes some solutions in his book, suggesting changing the current format to match structures that have been successful in other insurance industries, such as homeowners, auto, and life insurance. There are three major components to achieving this shift.[16]

1. Each person would be required to purchase catastrophic health insurance to cover true catastrophes in one's health from birth to grave. With everyone contributing to this insurance pool, and the majority not needing to use it, the rate would be affordable. These plans would have a $25,000–$30,000 deductible, so would be used only for catastrophic illnesses or accidents.

2. Everyone also would have a mandatory health savings account (HSA). This account would have tax incentives and be used for all routine healthcare. All would be responsible

for their own health and what is spent on their care. Their HSA would come from their own money; there would be no third-party payers. Users would become the true consumers. This could create a welcome competition in pricing, quality, and transparency of healthcare services.

3. If people have an unforeseen illness or health challenge that exceeds the money in their current health savings account, they would have the option to borrow against their future HSA contributions. In this way, healthcare costs could be managed even for unforeseen events with a loan that would not impact their personal operating budget.

These changes would require a fundamental shift in education, attitude, and understanding about healthcare costs and current healthcare insurance. People are led to believe they could never afford to cover the cost of usual and customary healthcare. But what most Americans do not realize is how much they are truly paying. It's a lot more than meets the eye, with just monthly premiums, deductibles, and out of pocket co-insurance amounts. There are the hidden costs such as capped salaries, so employers can pay for rising healthcare costs. Also, remember that nearly 20 percent of your federal income tax and 10 percent of your state income tax goes toward financing healthcare.

Let's look at an example that Goldhill outlines in detail in his book:[17]

Becky

Becky is a new employee whose annual salary is $35,000. What she does not realize is that when a company budgets a new position, the benefits that the company must pay for each

160

employee are factored into the salary. While the collective cost to the company, including her benefits, is $43,000, her salary is adjusted for those benefits, and she is offered $35,000. While her portion of the annual medical premiums is only $2,112, with tax and Social Security deductions, her net pay is only $25,107. Here is an example of her pay stub:

SALARY	$35,000
Taxes State, $1,276 Federal, $3,827 Social Security, $2,170 Medicare, $508	-$7,781
Other deductions Medical, $1932 Dental, $114 Vision, $66	-$2112
NET PAY	$25,107

But wait . . . what is Becky truly paying for her healthcare? Besides the obvious costs of her premiums and deductibles, there are disguised costs that Becky is contributing to fund healthcare.

Let's look further.

Medicare Part A—Becky pays $508. But her employer also pays $508 that doesn't show up on her pay stub. In effect, her Medicare contribution is $1016.	$1016
20% of $3827 federal income tax paid by Becky—directed to healthcare	$765

10% of $1276 state income tax paid by Becky—directed to health care	$128
Don't forget her deductible	$35
And that she's bearing the brunt of her compensation burden (Remember her salary is quoted as $35,000, but her true compensation, from the company's perspective, is $43,000, including benefits and employer taxes. This figure represents the amount the company is paying for her healthcare benefits.)	$5,679
Her annual medical, vision and dental insurance premiums	$2,112
Total visible and hidden costs that Becky and her company paid on her behalf. (This represents more than 23% of her true gross income of $43,000.)	$10,050

Excerpted from *Catastrophic Care: Why Everything We Think We Know about Health Care Is Wrong* and used with permission from David Goldhill.

Most Americans, like Becky, have no idea what they actually pay for healthcare annually. In Goldhill's book, he continues the Becky scenario to illustrate what she might pay for healthcare over her lifetime, assuming that she marries, has two children, stays relatively healthy, works until age 65, and dies at age 80. Though hypothetical, he demonstrates that she could spend upwards of 40–50 percent of her lifetime income on healthcare costs including direct and hidden costs.

What is it going to take to convince Americans that this system is not working? Are there any other businesses that you would support that continue to be more expensive, yet provide less care and sub-optimal results and become more fragmented and dysfunctional by the year? According to the American Psychological Association poll on stress released November 1, 2017, the top stressor for 43 percent of Americans is healthcare.[18] We must do something to change this.

Collectively, Americans are paying $2.5 trillion annually for healthcare. It's estimated that 25 percent of this is wasted on administrative costs due to a complex third-party insurer billing system requiring more staff and time to manage. Do we really want to continue paying such large amounts into a system that values sickness, expanded use of services, and health insurers shareholders' profits more than the health, wellness, and vitality of Americans?

More and more horror stories are emerging regarding which services are covered and which are not. Here are some examples: One patient was scheduled to have surgery in her local hospital. When she investigated to see what her insurance company would cover, she learned that her hospitalization and surgeon's bill would be covered, but the anesthesia would not be a covered service. Apparently, the anesthesiology group with that particular hospital did not have a contract with her insurance company. This was disturbing to me to think that a surgery would be covered but not the anesthesia services.

Another patient was a diver while in high school and suffered an injury to his right shoulder. Last year when he applied for health insurance, he was quoted a rate that would include a $2,500 deductible. However, it included a clause for a $10,000 deductible for anything involving his right shoulder. This is a travesty for a 28-year-old. Clearly, major changes are desperately needed.

By creating healthcare savings accounts, the money paid into the healthcare system would come directly from consumers. Third-party payer costs, concerns about their profit margins, and wasteful, ineffective administrative costs would be eliminated. Additionally, if people are direct consumers of healthcare, costs would become much more transparent. This would drive competitive pricing, which ultimately decreases costs, similar to what has happened in every other industry. The indirect effect for providers would be more direct time spent with patients since they would no longer need to use 30 percent of their energy and resources for billing and insurance management—greatly benefiting providers and consumers.

Currently there is very little transparency in healthcare. Most hospitals, laboratories, and medical equipment companies cannot tell you what a product, test, or service will cost because it depends on the contract between your insurance company and the provider. In many cases, even when medically indicated, it is not apparent which tests and services insurance companies will cover until they are billed.

Here is a recent example. My husband had his annual labs done through my office and billed through his Anthem insurance. He had a vitamin D level tested since his previous level was low and he regularly takes a vitamin D supplement. We live in Louisville, Kentucky, but his health insurance is provided by Iowa Blue Cross and Blue Shield Anthem, since his employer's parent company is in Dubuque, Iowa. In Kentucky, the local Anthem Blue Cross and Blue Shield insurance company covers vitamin D levels. However, the Iowa Anthem did not cover the vitamin D test. Iowa Anthem's explanation of benefits showed that the test was not covered due to lack of medical necessity.

I sent the insurance company his medical records, which documented the necessity for testing his vitamin D level, and yet it was still denied. When I spoke to the representative, she told me, "Not a day goes by that someone doesn't ask me why we don't cover vitamin D tests." What was extremely frustrating is that the vitamin D test was billed by the laboratory that ran the test for $232. Our office account's bill rate with the same company for a vitamin D level is $42. How much does it really cost? Is it $42 or $232? Reluctantly, we paid the $232 to Quest for the test. This is an example of why transparency in healthcare services is needed.

Transparency would be a natural consequence if all Americans were using healthcare savings accounts. Not only would transparency drive competition, but also consumers would know exactly what they are expected to pay for a desired service before it is completed. The cost for tests and services will be actual fees for a service instead of a grossly inflated rate that is common in healthcare industries.

Another positive consequence of our managing our healthcare spending is that we will be encouraged to take more responsibility for our health and well-being. No longer will the overriding perception be that our healthcare is dependent on a third-party health insurance company. In my integrative practice, we do not participate with insurance providers. Our practice model of wellness and disease prevention does not fit into the current disease-care insurance-based structure. We operate as a cash-based practice. Naturally, a common question asked by many people who call to inquire about our services is whether their insurance will cover our services. Many people have the perception that if their insurance company doesn't cover a service, then they cannot have it, regardless of how beneficial it might be. Yet, our services are available for all. Using individual health savings accounts would eliminate this perception.

Increasing individual responsibility for health through health savings accounts will promote wellness and disease prevention. The current disease-care model encourages people to wait until they are really sick before seeking healthcare. If people become more accountable and responsible for their individual health, a stronger focus would be placed on wellness and disease prevention. People know that an ounce of prevention is worth a pound of cure, and if they are responsible for their own health savings accounts, they will be more likely to seek preventive care. Also, they will be able to use their funds for creating optimal health instead of wasting a significant amount for insurance premiums.

In the event that an unforeseen illness or health challenge arises, they would pay for needed health services through their healthcare savings account. If the money in their health savings account is insufficient to cover the costs of an operation or procedure, they could borrow from their future health savings contributions. These healthcare costs would not come from their daily operating budget. These costs, therefore, would not cause medical bankruptcy.

In Goldhill's example, it is clear that we are paying much more for healthcare beyond insurance premiums, deductibles, and co-payments. If everyone funded their individual health savings account, they would have the money to cover costs of unforeseen illnesses. The direct consumer process would foster competition and transparency to help lower costs for surgeries and procedures, thus making these affordable and able to be financed through individual health savings accounts.

People have asked what would happen if a person has an unexpectedly large bill. Remember that each person would be required to purchase catastrophic health insurance, which would be applicable to healthcare bills in excess of $25,000. Some also have wondered about those who are unable to afford a health savings account or catastrophic health insurance. This model would replace third-party insurers. It would not replace Medicare or Medicaid. However, with the added transparency and direct fee for service, competition would drive down all medical costs, including the medical costs for Medicare and Medicaid.

Goldhill's ideas would radically reform how Americans finance healthcare. It's time to put the responsibility into the hands of the actual consumers of health—without the surrogates. As he admits, a change of this magnitude might take a couple of generations, but we owe it to ourselves, our health, our financial well-being, our children's health and well-being, and our providers' health and well-being to begin the shift now.

What about providers? Many are experiencing increased barriers to their practice. Hospitals and insurers are demanding that providers see an increased number of patients in shorter appointment times and yet maintain a high quality of care. Many physicians are choosing to leave conventional medicine or worse yet, stop practicing medicine all together. Here is how a young doctor described the current healthcare climate and her frustrations with the system.[19]

Dear Hippocrates,

I want a divorce.

Let's face it, you and I were young, idealistic, and naive when we met. Everyone said we were "perfect for each other," valedictorian and humanitarian. We thought we could change the world, one sacrifice at a time. Sleep deprivation, grueling academic hurdles, delayed gratification. We proudly wore those badges as a testament to our commitment together when we started our board-certified family medicine profession in 2003.

I should've signed a pre-nup.

Slowly, the tendrils of distrust curled around our world. Insurance didn't trust our decision-making, so formularies became a paradoxical, rigid moving target. Patients wouldn't trust our recommendations, certain that their latest Google search was far more medically sound. Hospital administration stopped trusting. Our world became a time and date-stamped arena, visible to all, helpful to none. Once a pillar of scientific benevolence, doctors were now stripped of power and treated with public skepticism.

To rein in this metastatic distrust, you suggested we collect and curate data. Surely, this would "improve" our nation's floundering healthcare system, right?! Never mind the suicidal grandfather in Room 3 . . . but did he agree to get his colonoscopy and tetanus updated?! Who cares if the basal cell skin cancer was recognized and treated on Mrs. Jones, did she sign up for a mammogram?! My resentment grew with each step into this minefield of check boxes.

This wasn't the life I planned for us. The inequality felt oppressive. I gazed longingly at our neighbors: The Specialists. Their grassy-green lives appeared unfettered by regulations because they could just advise, "Follow up with your primary care doctor. They'll take care of it all."

But I couldn't.

Your expectations of our relationship had morphed into something unrecognizable. Gone were the moments I hoped to bask in the glow of empathy, caring, and healing. Do you recall the vows we took, Hippocrates? "I will remember that there is art to medicine as well as science, and that warmth, sympathy, and understanding may outweigh the surgeon's knife or the chemist's drug."

A far cry from your modern version. Today's words are icily brisk as we shiver past each other in the crowded hallways. You speak in modifiers, ICD-10 codes, and triplicate forms. My Love Languages are Touch and Words. Yours is EMR. Your eyes practically glow brighter than the screen when a new data collection feature is unveiled, lengthening the nurse's duties from 15 to 20 minutes for each patient check-in. It's obvious you love to flirt with inefficiency.

You shift the boundaries of our relationship on a daily basis, expecting me to jump through unnecessary hoops against the backdrop of "more patient access." How can I detect the insidious hemochromatosis or educate the infertile polycystic patient when I'm interrupted with your ridiculous demands to answer every message or refill with neck-breaking speed?

First, do no harm . . . correct?

Yet, I continued to adapt my workflow to be more efficient, clinging to the knowledge that if I didn't care, who would? I work harder, you pay me less. (Even less as a female physician.) And now all we do is fight over money, when we really should be fighting over the real downfall of us: your adultery. When you stepped out and had an affair with Press Ganey [a leading provider of patient satisfaction surveys], you changed the tapestry of our relationship forever.

In your shortsighted effort to measure value based on antiquated patient satisfaction scores, you adeptly placed my vitality and compassion in hospice. How can my worth be stripped down to a number, when I'm pressured to see more volume, squeezing as much as I can in 15 minutes? I feel underappreciated, and I deserve better.

It's not about the money, Hippocrates. It never was. No matter how many miles I run, sun salutations I cycle through, or glasses of wine I sip, I decided:

We have become incompatible.

Our core values have diverged so far apart, it's impossible to reconcile our differences. Despite the tone of this letter, I am not angry; I'm disappointed. However, I'm filled more with gratitude for our chapter together. Relationships aren't measured in time, but rather the amount of growth and meaning. Because of you, I have an amazing skill set, memories to fill my heart, and a clear foundation to pursue my next passion . . . customizable to my definitions.

In the end, only three things matter: how much you loved, how gently you lived, and how gracefully you let go of things not meant for you. —Buddha

Best wishes,

Your American Family Doctor

P.S.—You can keep my stethoscope, but please return my boxed set of *The Walking Dead*. The moment those zombies hit, I'll volunteer to be everyone's Hershel.

—Lara Salyer Smith, MD

Reprinted with permission by Lara Salyer Smith, MD, founder of Health Innate clinic, healthin8.com, in Green County, Wisconsin, where she practices functional medicine.

So, who does the current healthcare system actually benefit? Certainly not providers, nor millions of Americans whose "healthcare" costs have increased while their services have decreased. It seems the only beneficiaries of the current system are the "health" insurance providers, hospitals, and healthcare service providers such as laboratories and durable medical equipment companies. It is time for a change.

---

1. Calculated from data from the United States Census Bureau, "Statistical Abstract of the US: 1989," US Census Bureau website, https://www.census. gov/library/publications/1989/compendia/statab/109ed.html; Enotes.com; the National Coalition on Health Care website, https://nchc.org/; the Kaiser Family Foundation website, https://www.kff.org/; and the Centers for Medicare and Medicaid Services, "National Health Expenditure Data," Centers for

Medicare and Medicaid Services website, www.cms.gov/Research-Statistics-Data-and-Systems/Statistics-Trends-and-Reports/NationalHealthExpendData/NationalHealthAccountsHistorical.html.

2. Centers for Medicare and Medicaid Services, "Research Statistics."

3. US Census, "Statistical Abstract, 1989"; Enotes.com; National Coalition on Health Care website; Kaiser Family Foundation website; and Centers for Medicare and Medicaid Services, "National Health Expenditures."

4. Centers for Medicare and Medicaid Services, "Research Statistics."

5. Weil, A, *Why Our Health Matters*, 2009.

6. David Goldhill, "How American Healthcare Killed My Father," *The Atlantic.* September 2009, https://www.theatlantic.com/magazine/archive/2009/09/how-american-health-care-killed-my-father/307617/, accessed October 23, 2017.

7. David Goldhill, *Catastrophic Care: Why Everything We Think We Know about Healthcare Is Wrong* (New York: First Vintage Books, 2013).

8. United Health Group, "Unitedhealth Group Reports 2016 Results Highlighted by Continued Strong and Diversified Growth," United Health Group website, https://unitedhealthgroup.com/content/dam/UHG/PDF/investors/2016/UNH-Q4-2016-Release.pdf, accessed October 23, 2017.

9. "Anthem Revenue, Profits: ANTM Annual Income Statement," Amigo Bulls website, https://amigobulls.com/stocks/ANTM/income-statement/annual, accessed October 23, 2017.

10. "Cigna Revenue, Profits: CI Annual Income Statement," Amigo Bulls website, https://amigobulls.com/stocks/CI/income-statement/annual, accessed October 23, 2017.

11. Aetna Company, "Aetna Reports Fourth-Quarter and Full-Year 2016 Results," Aetna website, https://news.aetna.com/news-releases/aetna-reports-fourth-quarter-and-full-year-2016-results/, accessed October 23, 2017.

12. "Humana Revenue, Profits: HUM Annual Income Statement," Amigo Bulls website, https://amigobulls.com/stocks/HUM/income-statement/annual, accessed October 23, 2017.

13. Leslie Small, "Health Insurance CEO Pay Tops Out at $17.3M in 2015," April 24, 2016, Fierce Healthcare website, https://www.fiercehealthcare.com/payer/health-insurance-ceo-pay-at-big-five-tops-out-at-17-3m-2015.

14. Patrick Kennedy, "CEO Pay Watch: UnitedHealth's Stephen Hemsley Made $31.3 Million Last Year," April 24, 2017, http://www.startribune.com/ceo-pay-watch-unitedhealth-s-stephen-hemsley-made-31-3-million-last-year/420284643/.

15. Goldhill, *Catastrophic Care.*

16. Ibid.

17. Ibid.

18. American Psychological Association, "Stress in America: The State of Our Nation," November 1, 2017. American Psychological Association website, http://www.apa.org/news/press/releases/stress/2017/state-nation.pdf.

19. Lara Salyer, "Dear Hippocrates: I Want a Divorce," August 13, 2016, Kevin MD website, https://www.kevinmd.com/blog/2016/08/dear-hippocrates-want-divorce.html.

CHAPTER 10

Transforming Healthcare: Healing You, Me, and Our Broken Disease-Care System

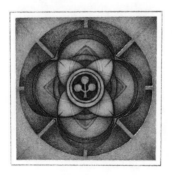

The Chinese word for crisis is composed of two characters, commonly translated as danger and opportunity. A more accurate translation is "critical point."[1] All three descriptors precisely describe where our broken disease-care system is today. We have truly reached a critical point where change is inevitable, desirable, and greatly needed. In the face of this crisis, we have enormous opportunity to transform healthcare into a system that works for everyone—providers and patients—and that is economically feasible.

We can begin transforming healthcare by shifting to patient-centric models, based on a culture of caring and compassion. This must begin at the top of an organization with strong leadership to create a collective vision and unified purpose of putting the patient first, no matter what. Next, words (such as hospital mission and vision statements) and actions must be aligned. The advertised slogan of one hospital in which I was employed was "Family Spoken Here." These were powerful words, but the hospital operated in an autocratic biomedical model and I commonly observed that the hospital and staff's needs took precedence over patients and families' needs.

Let's revisit the example of the visitation (pun intended) policy in the intensive care unit of this hospital. Despite ample research validating the benefits to patients and family members for open visitation in critical care units, some staff would not allow families to visit their loved ones. In some cases, the staff had the perception that families would be in the way of their care delivery. Further investigation found that sometimes these nurses were simply easily intimidated by families, had poor communication skills, or were insecure about their nursing skills. In these instances, they put their own needs (albeit not always consciously) above the patients' and families' needs. The hospital vision and mission statement—Family Spoken Here—became empty words.

Another local hospital has used this advertising slogan throughout the city, "Aggressive Treatment, Compassionate Care." While this hospital is beginning to heed the desires of patients to create systems based on an integrative medicine philosophy, it's with a catch. The hospital is piloting integrative medicine on one floor of their newly remodeled women and children's hospital. Patients on this floor can experience aromatherapy, Reiki, or massage. However, the staff members who provide Reiki or massage therapy have to deliver these on their own time as volunteers. Compassionate care must be afforded to everyone—not just patients and family, but also staff. It's unreasonable to expect that professionals will deliver valuable patient care on a volunteer basis. Again, the words and actions of this hospital's advertisement are inconsistent.

A culture of whole-person healing must be supported by the entire organization. Otherwise it risks the words and actions not being aligned. Lucia Thornton, in *Whole Person Caring: An Interprofessional Model for Healing and Wellness*, beautifully articulates the comparison of traditional biomedical models and whole-person caring models.[2] (See table.)[3]

Comparison of Models of Health Care Practice

Current Biomedical Model	Model of Whole-Person Caring
People are seen primarily as biological (bio-psycho-social) beings.	People are seen primarily as spiritual (sacred) beings.
Focus is on physical/physiological symptoms and illness.	Focus is on nourishing a person's wholeness (body-mind-heart-soul).
Focus is on diagnosis and treatment of disease.	Focus is on promoting healthy lifestyle practices.
Emphasis is on cure.	Emphasis is on healing/harmony.
Emphasis is on suppression and/or relief of symptoms.	Emphasis is on exploring meaning and source of symptoms.
Illness seen as negative, something to fix.	Illness is seen as an opportunity to explore and shift lifestyle patterns.

The professional is the authority, the one in charge.	The professional is a therapeutic partner.
The professional is emotionally neutral.	The professional's caring is an important component of healing.
The patient is encouraged to rely on the professional for health care needs.	The person is empowered and encouraged to promote his or her own health.
Hierarchical relationships are valued and encouraged.	Nonhierarchical relationships are valued and encouraged; shared governance is the norm.
The professional orchestrates care.	Patient-professional collaboration is welcomed.

Reprinted with permission, ©2013 by Lucia Thornton, *Whole Person Caring: An Interprofessional Model for Healing and Wellness.*

Together we can create a healthcare system that is truly patient-centric (whole-person centered) with the best interests of the patient and family first and foremost. Imagine what such a system looks like.

In patient-centric, whole-person centered models, the systems operationalize health and wholeness not only for patients and families, but also for individual staff and the organization. Let's explore what this would mean.

In a patient-centric model, care for patients and families will not only meet physical and physiologic needs but also include emotional, psychological, and spiritual aspects of healing. A common psychological concept taught in most health-related curricula is Abraham Maslow's famous Hierarchy of Needs.[4]

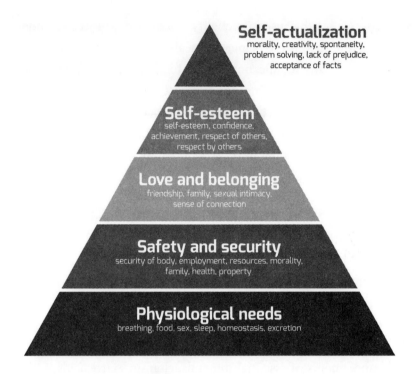

Maslow's Hierarchy of Needs

His five-tier model of human beings' needs is depicted on a pyramid that includes basic physiologic needs (breathing, food, water, and sleep) as the first tier, and progresses to self-actualization as the top tier. As elemental and necessary as the first-tier needs are, they are often slighted (especially food and sleep) and even abused for some patients and families in hospital environments.

In patient-centric models, all providers acknowledge the healing and restoration that occurs during sleep and will prioritize the timing of treatments and tests to ensure that patients and families are allowed at least six to eight hours of uninterrupted sleep.

Food service is a basic example within a truly patient-centric institution where everything, including finances, is subordinate to the best interests of the patient.[5] Many hospitals contract to provide meals from companies that use low-quality, inexpensive, processed foods. Knowing that food is medicine, the meals served in a patient-centric model are healthy, organic, non-GMO foods without pesticides and preservatives, even if that means a higher cost to the hospital.

Processed foods and those that have been genetically modified are eliminated. The food that is served is prepared with love and an intention to bring healing to those who will be consuming it. Meals are planned, not only to nourish patients and families, but also to teach them the benefits of a healthy, predominately plant-based diet.

Some hospitals have even created organic gardens to grow vegetables, produce, and herbs used for preparing food for patients and staff. Hospitals are beginning to partner with local farmers to provide locally grown fruit, vegetables, and herbs. Local farmers may also provide eggs from free-range chickens and organic beef and chicken, raised without the use of antibiotics or growth hormones. To support daily nutritional needs, patients could be provided with daily supplements of essential minerals, vitamins, fatty acids, amino acids, and probiotics.

The next tier in Maslow's hierarchy is safety and security. In a patient-centric model, safety is a top initiative of the hospital. Not only is it safe for a nurse, physician, therapist, or other employee to point out any potential safety issues, it is encouraged. As mentioned earlier, if errors occur in patient care delivery, these are evaluated as a breach of the system and not as an opportunity for disciplinary measures or to scapegoat one employee. Each occurrence is systematically evaluated to see where safety measures of the system can be improved or changed to enhance staff efficacy and most importantly, patient outcomes. This attitude toward errors facilitates trust and an "I've got your back" culture, with everyone working for the common good of the patient and family. Evidence-based protocols are instituted system-wide when proven to improve patient outcomes.

The top three tiers of Maslow's hierarchy are often overlooked or overshadowed by the physical needs in conventional medicine. In a patient-centric model, emphasis is placed on body, mind, heart, and soul. Staff takes time to be totally present with patients, allowing them to express their feelings and perhaps explore the deeper meaning or purpose of their illness.

Simply rubbing a patient's back with lotion, freshening their sheets, or fluffing their pillows are small acts of compassion that can greatly enhance a patient's healing and well-being. Providers can focus on methods to make patients more comfortable in addition to alleviating their pain or suffering. Many patient-centric organizations include therapies such as massage, Reiki, art therapy, and aromatherapy to further enhance patients' healing and well-being.

In patient-centric models, the patient and family are the primary focus. Physicians, nurses, and other care providers are partners in their health. This emphasis creates a two-way dialogue instead of the predominant provider-directed conversation. In the integrative medicine fellowship I undertook at the University of Arizona, we were trained in motivational interviewing. This practice involves beginning with the patients' goals for health, determining what strategies have worked toward improving their health, and together establishing health goals. This is much different from the authoritarian structure of the patient being a passive recipient of the healthcare provider's orders. There is richness in the dialogue between patients and providers that is equally beneficial for both. Patients gain trust that their opinions are important and are therefore more likely to divulge information that could be critical to their health goals. This information may even change the provider's original plan of care. Providers are equally benefited by a more fulfilling personal relationship with patients. Once healthcare goals are mutually established, providers do the following to help patients attain their healthcare goals:

- Hold patients accountable

- Help them identify and overcome unforeseen obstacles

- Modify the treatment plan when necessary

All members of the team in a patient-centric model— physicians, nurses, therapists, and nursing assistants—work together in an interdisciplinary approach for the good of patients and families. Each team member is recognized as a vital part of the team and acknowledged for their unique talents, expertise, and individual contributions to the care of the patient. There is no imbalance of power or control. Each person is respected as a worthy and important member of the patient care team. There is zero tolerance for disruptive behaviors of any kind. Patient-centric models shift the culture of fear, frustration, and burnout to one of compassion, caring, and healthy behaviors. There is an overlying atmosphere of joy, satisfaction, teamwork, and camaraderie prevalent throughout the system.

This culture of compassion is also extended to providers. Nurses are encouraged to work to the full extent of their licensure. They are trained to use holistic modalities to enhance patients' well-being such as healing touch, Reiki, and aromatherapy. They acknowledge the profound value of creating a healing environment based on listening and supporting patients and families. They have time built into their day to take five to ten minutes to evaluate patients' needs using comfort scales. The nurses support each other. If one nurse is having a particularly intense day, colleagues are there to help, knowing that on another day, they might be the ones who need an extra hand. Nursing staff is afforded support in order to take time for meals and breaks from patient care delivery. Many hospitals have created a yoga or meditation room in which staff can take a break, relax, and rejuvenate to maintain their energy to continue to provide excellent care and compassion for patients. Self-care is encouraged and supported.

Following are three idealized patient scenarios to further illustrate patient-centric, whole-person care delivery models.

Cindy

Cindy is 54 and has recently discovered a pea-sized lump in her left breast. She is distraught and realizes the timing of this discovery could not be worse. She reflects on how tumultuous the last two years have been while enduring a painful divorce. She is just now getting her life back together. She has moved to a new home, begun a new job, and has had to manage not only her own emotions surrounding the divorce, but also support her two teenage daughters with all the abrupt changes in their lives. She fears that one of her daughters is using drugs and alcohol to cope with all the changes.

As Cindy walks into St. Mary's Hospital, she fears the worst. She heads to the radiology department for her mammogram. She signs in and sits in the waiting room. Michelle, the X-ray technician greets her to take her back for her mammogram. Michelle notices that Cindy appears tense and nervous, then asks her, "Are you okay?"

With that, Cindy breaks into tears and tells Michelle that she is very afraid of having breast cancer. Michelle hugs her and holds her for a moment allowing Cindy to cry. Michelle encourages her to breathe and asks if there is anything else she can do for her. Cindy asks Michelle if she would mind saying a prayer for her. Michelle says she would be happy to.

Cindy relaxes and proceeds to have her mammogram. Divine intervention just provided a compassionate, caring X-ray technician for her to do her mammogram. Cindy realizes this breast lump could be a wake-up call for her to focus on her own health and well-being and knows that she must make some healthier choices in order to create her optimal health of mind, body, and spirit.

The mammogram does confirm a mass and she is referred to an oncologist, Dr. Matthew, who performs a biopsy and confirms that Cindy has stage II estrogen-receptor positive adenocarcinoma. Dr. Matthew acknowledges that he knows she is scared and assures her that he is part of a clinic that uses a team approach to help patients through their treatment and recovery process. Cindy is touched by his kindness and sincerity.

Dr. Matthew introduces Cindy to Maria, a nurse practitioner in the clinic. Maria meets with Cindy to review the next steps for her treatment and address her main immediate concerns. Cindy shares that she is very worried about the cancer diagnosis, the possibility of surgery, chemotherapy, and radiation. She is fearful about who will care for her daughters if something happens to her and shares the events of the last two years. Maria says that she would like to set up a patient care conference for her the next week with all the key members of her team. Maria states that besides Dr. Matthew and herself, the team will include a nutritionist, a counselor, and a chaplain for spiritual support. Maria adds that they have several team members to provide stress management therapies including Reiki, massage, HeartMath®, and art therapy. She asks Cindy if she is interested in any of these in her treatment plan. Cindy says that, although she sees a massage therapist about once a month, she still feels overwhelmed with stress. She has also heard about HeartMath® and how beneficial it can be for stress reduction. Maria adds Kimberly, the HeartMath® provider and life coach, to Cindy's team and encourages her to invite her massage therapist to the care conference the following week.

Maria makes a list of Cindy's questions regarding therapy options, survival rates, and typical recovery for the potential treatment regimens. Maria will share these questions with the team, so they can be prepared to review them with her. Maria encourages Cindy to bring her mother, sister, daughters, and whoever else will be supporting her through her healing process to their meetings. Cindy is relieved that she can bring her best friend, Tracy.

The patient care conference held the following week is very successful. Dr. Matthew presents the advantages and disadvantages of all the treatment options. Other team members contribute their expertise to Cindy's care plan. Cindy feels supported, guided, and confident in the treatment plan to have a mastectomy with reconstruction of her left breast. Her surgery is scheduled for the next week. Before she leaves the clinic, she meets with Dr. Youngson, an anesthesiologist, to review instructions for her upcoming surgery. She has heard horror stories about surgical consent forms and is pleasantly surprised when she reads this one and appreciative that it has been given to her a week in advance of her surgery. This allows her time to read the consent form while in a relaxed state and be afforded time to ask any questions. The consent form reads:

On October 10, 2017, you will have a mastectomy of your left breast to be performed by Dr. Matthew. I, Dr. Youngson, will administer your anesthesia. We are part of a highly trained compassionate team that will treat you. In rare instances (less than 2 percent), things don't go as planned. Please know that our staff has received special training to act in these emergent situations. We will do everything possible to ensure that you are well cared for and remain comfortable. If there is something we can do to enhance your comfort, please let us know.

Cindy asks if she can bring headphones so she can listen to relaxing music and her loving-kindness meditation. Dr. Youngson agrees that would be a great idea.

Cindy has her surgery the following week and everything goes well. She was grateful to have met with Kimberly a few days before her surgery, as the HeartMath® techniques proved to be extremely beneficial in helping her manage her anxiety. Her lymph nodes were all negative and the tumor had very clear margins. She has reconstructive surgery a few weeks after her mastectomy and will continue taking tamoxifen for five years. She is ever grateful to her team. Her body heals quickly. With the help of the nutritionist, she is eating a much healthier diet and is exercising four to five days a week. The counselor not only helps Cindy, but also intervened with one of Cindy's daughters, who experienced her own wake-up call with her mother's breast cancer diagnosis.

Would this be an accurate illustration of care delivered in your hospital or clinic? Though hypothetical, there are currently facilities that use patient-centered models or are beginning to use a whole-person approach. Keith Block, MD, is an integrative oncologist who founded the Block Center for Integrative Cancer Treatment in Skokie, Illinois, in 1980.[6] In his center, patients receive individualized integrative approaches to nutrition, mind-body therapies, exercise, and supplements, along with conventional cancer treatments to achieve the best outcomes. These types of clinics are inspiring and reflective of how systems can be implemented based on whole-person models of care.

Len Saputo, MD, is board certified in internal medicine and is the founder of the Health Medicine Center in Walnut Creek, California, which uses a multidisciplinary team to provide individualized care for patients. For patients with complex chronic illnesses from which successful outcomes have not been achieved with conventional medicine, a healing circle process is used. Patients meet with a health guide (usually their primary care provider) to see which practitioners would be appropriate to invite to their circle given the patient's clinical needs. Patients are asked to put in writing what they hope to gain from the circle experience.

The circle includes the patient and three to eight practitioners from a variety of disciplines. The group meets for approximately two hours. After introductions, patients begin by sharing their health issues and what they hope to gain from the circle experience. Next, each practitioner discusses suggestions and possible interventions to benefit the patient. When complete, a brief post-healing circle meeting is continued without the patient to coordinate the final treatment plan.

Here are some of the benefits patients derive from healing circles:[7]

- Practical information is given to help resolve patients' illnesses from the viewpoint of several disciplines.

- Patients are empowered and supported to explore psycho-spiritual issues, i.e., the deeper meaning of their illness.

- From the group interconnectedness, a shift often occurs from information exchange to profound healing.

Dr. Saputo describes that through this interconnectedness and heightened awareness, deeper insight into the spiritual meaning of illness is revealed. An ideal strategic approach most suitable for the situation emerges from the collective wisdom of the group.[8] The use of healing circles is truly an effective tool within patient-centric, whole-person models of healthcare.

Let's explore another patient scenario illustrated through Mark's story.

Mark

"Hey, Mark. It's a beautiful day. Let's go play golf!" yells Mark's next-door neighbor, Rick. Mark loves playing golf and knows that it would be a great way to reduce the stress he's recently experienced stemming from his executive position at the bank.

"Great idea, Rick. Let me check with Carol."

Mark then returns from the house. "Let's go!"

On the way to the golf course, Mark notices an epigastric pain in his chest and thinks to himself, "That breakfast must not be settling so well." Rick notices that Mark is sweating and somewhat pale. "Are you feeling all right, man?"

Mark answers, "It must be something I ate for breakfast."

They load up their clubs and head to the first hole to tee off. Rick notices that Mark is short of breath and still sweating quite a bit. The first two holes go well. Both men feel as if they are "on their game."

Then, just as Mark starts to tee off on the third hole, he clutches his chest and collapses. Rick immediately begins CPR and yells to another golfer to call 911. By a stroke of luck, an ambulance happens to be near the golf course and, within minutes, two EMTs are on the scene. They bring a defibrillator and shock Mark's heart. After two shocks, Mark is conscious and says he feels as if an elephant is standing on his chest. The EMTs determine he is having a heart attack and quickly get him into the ambulance to take him to the nearest hospital.

Rick calls Carol to tell her what has happened, and she hurriedly drives to meet Mark at St. Francis Hospital. Several thoughts are going through her mind. Is Mark going to die? He had been complaining that all of the pressure from work was creating a lot of anxiety for him. Carol had noticed that Mark had been having frequent indigestion lately, and now wonders if his pain was actually heart-related.

Carol finds Mark in room 9 of the emergency department. The doctor is reviewing his electrocardiogram and has already contacted a cardiologist. After conferring with the cardiologist, they agree that Mark needs an immediate cardiac catheterization to evaluate his heart circulation.

The cardiologist determines that Mark's left anterior descending artery has a 95 percent blockage and will need a stent to open it. After the procedure is completed, Mark admits that he feels much better and realizes that for the first time in a long while, he can take a deep breath without a nagging persistent ache just under his breastbone. The cardiologist tells him how lucky he is that Rick knew how to do CPR and that the EMTs were so near.

Lying on the table in the cardiac recovery area, Mark becomes aware that he must make some dramatic changes in his life. He realizes that life is short, and his family, health, and well-being mean more to him than any executive position. Carol joins him in the recovery area where he tells her that he has made the decision to resign from his position. Carol is greatly relieved. She knows that he has been offered other positions with comparable salaries and fewer stressors. Carol says, "Let's just focus on you for now and healing your heart."

Carol asks the nurse if the hospital offers any programs for people with heart disease. The nurse enthusiastically shares information on the APO E Gene Diet and exercise program. The nurse gives Carol *The Perfect Gene Diet* so she can learn more about the program. It turns out that the hospital has just begun a comprehensive cardiovascular health program including the APO E diet, exercise with a fitness trainer, yoga, meditation, and stress management. The hospital is currently enrolling patients for the program that will begin the following week. Mark can't help but marvel at the synchronicity of the program relative to what has happened to him. He admits to Carol that he saw his life flash before his eyes and feels certain that he is supposed to join this class. He adds that he thinks his heart needs to heal physically, emotionally, and spiritually, and that this program could provide healing in all those areas.

Many hospitals and facilities are recognizing the impact that healthy lifestyle management has on the incidence, prevention, and reversal of heart disease. Dean Ornish, MD, was one of the first physicians to demonstrate that heart disease is reversible. He has created a program called Reversing Heart Disease, which has been instituted in 23 centers across the country.[9] The tenets of his program are nutrition, group therapy, stress management, and fitness.

Pamela McDonald, author of *The Perfect Gene Diet*, has created an online version of her APO E Gene Diet program including the ability to locate a trained provider in various areas.[10]

Here is a third scenario to illustrate patient-centric models in the clinic setting.

Terri

Terri has just developed a cold and upper respiratory illness. She is a teacher's aide and remembers one of the students being sent home a couple of days before with a fever, cough, and head congestion. Terri's husband, Jim, suggests that she go to his employer's recently created onsite medical clinic. The clinic treats acute illnesses and also focuses on disease prevention for employees and their family members. After a couple days pass and Terri still does not feel well, she agrees to seek help.

Upon entering the clinic, she is impressed by the warm inviting décor. The registration area is pale blue, promoting a calm, serene feeling. There are live plants on either side of the waiting area. A beautiful oak table in the middle of the room holds a perpetual fountain, featuring running water over a rock bed. Terri is greeted immediately by the receptionist and offered a cup of ginger peach tea. She signs in and her name is called within minutes.

The medical assistant, Andrea, introduces herself and thanks Terri for coming to the clinic. Andrea tells Terri that since it is her first visit, she will have the full 60-minute consult with Dr. Melinda. Terri's first thought is, Wow! Typically, I wait an hour and am seen by the doctor for less than 15 minutes. Here I waited less than 15 minutes and will be seen for an hour.

Dr. Melinda does a thorough examination and asks Terri how she had previously managed her cold and flu symptoms. Dr. Melinda suggests that she:

- Increase her daily vitamin C intake to 4000–5000 milligrams a day for one week

- Double the probiotic that she was using for one week

- Take ViraClear three times daily to shorten the duration of her upper respiratory symptoms

- Take two Sinus Blend tablets two to three times daily to help keep her sinuses uncongested

Dr. Melinda also talks with Terri about using a Neti pot to help clear her sinuses. Terri feels relieved that Dr. Melinda didn't immediately jump to prescribing an antibiotic.

Next, Dr. Melinda asks Terri if she has any concerns about her overall health. Terri tells her that her menstrual cycles have become more irregular and that she is beginning to have occasional hot flashes. Also, her cholesterol level has begun to increase over the last year or so. Dr. Melinda suggests scheduling a future appointment to discuss hormone replacement. Terri tells Dr. Melinda that if she did any hormone replacement, she would prefer bio-identical hormones. Dr. Melinda tells her that she would be happy to accommodate her request for bio-identical hormones.

Dr. Melinda gives Terri a handout on the Mediterranean Diet and suggests that once Terri's symptoms improve, she increase her exercise to four to five times weekly. Terri leaves the clinic feeling much better. She is greatly impressed with the professionalism and thoroughness of her clinic visit.

Today companies and employers are seeking creative options to contain their healthcare expenditures in an attempt to reduce the overall healthcare costs for their employees. Activate Healthcare, in Indianapolis, is successfully helping businesses meet these goals. Their mission is to help transform healthcare by helping employees take charge of their health and employers take charge of healthcare costs.[11]

Activate Healthcare partners with businesses to help them contain healthcare expenditures by creating a wellness-focused culture within their organizations. Wellness clinics are created on site to support easy access for employees and their families. The clinics are provided as an additional health benefit for employees. Incentives are structured to promote wellness and disease prevention. Providers employed at the clinics are given tools to help support patients' health and well-being, such as nutrition guides, exercise regimens, and smoking cessation programs. Providers are afforded longer appointment times so a patient's chronic illnesses and complex health issues can be managed effectively. This structure not only promotes a high quality of healthcare delivery, but also provides a high degree of satisfaction for the provider and the employees.

One such example is the Plumbers & Steamfitters Local 440 Union, which has partnered with Activate Healthcare. A Health and Wellness Center was created on site and provides varying hours to accommodate employee work schedules. The clinic is open from six a.m. to four p.m. on Mondays and Wednesdays and from nine a.m. to six p.m. on Tuesdays and Thursdays. Friday hours are six a.m. to noon. A nurse is on call to accommodate anyone who needs care outside of regular operating hours. Initial patient visits are scheduled for 45 to 60 minutes, which affords the provider time to thoroughly address acute or chronic illnesses. For employee members, there is no cost for the office visits or for any generic prescriptions.

Partnerships such as this are the models of future healthcare clinics. The on-site clinics afford ease and convenience for employees to maintain good health, promoting a culture of vitality and well-being instead of the usual disease-care models.

Can you see from these examples just how healthcare can truly be transformed? The time to move these concepts from the hypothetical into reality is now—not just for a few clinics or hospitals but for all healthcare facilities in America. No longer can we remain oblivious to the emperor's lack of clothing and wait to intervene until people are sick. We must educate patients about healthy behaviors and empower them to take responsibility for their own health and well-being.

Hospital administrators must be courageous, persistent, and absolute in their resolve to create and support patient-centric, whole-person models based on patient safety and evidence-based practices in which nothing (including finances) is subordinate to the best interest of patients and families. Finally, all personnel, administrators, and providers must be models of health and well-being by continuing to improve their own health of mind, body, and spirit. As care providers, it is imperative that we model excellent health habits. It shows a lack of integrity to encourage patients to adopt healthy habits but not value our own health enough to practice what we preach. As providers, we often overlook self-care, yet it couldn't be more important. As the adage goes, actions speak louder than words. Our patients are watching and observing our actions!

You have made it to the end of this book. To help you continue your own journey toward wellness, I have included 10 simple daily tips, adopted from our Intentional Wellness Program that my colleagues and I developed in 2008. They are intended to help you achieve your optimal health of mind, body, and spirit.

Top 10 Daily Wellness Tips

1. Sleep seven to eight hours a night.

2. Go the extra smile.

3. Eat six servings of fruits and vegetables.

4.   Move your body joyfully.

5.   Connect with love.

6.   Feel gratitude in your heart and share it.

7.   Hydrate with clean water.

8.   Help someone.

9.   Be happy regardless.

10. Forgive and let go.

Now is the time for transforming healthcare and for healing our broken disease-care system. Let's create systems that we can each be proud of, and that we would feel confident and comforted to take our loved ones to for health and healing. Together, we can transform healthcare into systems of true healing, caring, compassion, wellness, and disease prevention. Let's do it! Our patients and families are counting on us to lead the way to optimal health and well-being for everyone.

------

1. Wikipedia, "Chinese Word for Crisis," https://en.wikipedia.org/wiki/Chinese_word_for_%22crisis%22, accessed October 23, 2017.

2. Lucia Thornton, *Whole Person Caring: An Interprofessional Model for Healing and Wellness* (Indianapolis: Sigma Theta Tau International, 2013).

3. Reprinted with permission from Lucia Thornton, *Whole Person Caring*.

4. Saul McLeod, "Maslow's Hierarchy of Needs," https://simplypsychology.org/maslow.html, accessed October 23, 2017.

5. Nance and Bartholomew, *Charting the Course*.

6. Keith Block, Block Center for Integrative Cancer Treatment, http://blockmd.com/, accessed October 23, 2017.

7. Len Saputo, *A Return to Healing: Radical Healthcare Reform and the Future of*

Medicine (San Rafael, CA: Origin Press, 2009).

8. Ibid.

9. Dean Ornish, *Dr. Dean Ornish's Program for Reversing Heart Disease: The Only System Scientifically Proven to Reverse Heart Disease without Drugs or Surgery* (New York: Random House, 1990).

10. McDonald, https://apoegenediet.com/.

11. Activate Healthcare, "Our Mission and Values," Activate Healthcare website, https://www.activatehealthcare.com/about-us/our-mission-and-values, accessed October 23, 2017.

Acknowledgments

I gratefully acknowledge the following people for their significant contribution in making this book possible:

Linda Eastman: Thank you for your patience and encouragement all along the way. You know that I carried parts of this book in my heart and mind for over 20 years. Finally, you were the inspiration and encouragement that I needed to bring it to fruition. I love you dearly.

Katherine Mapother: Your comments and edits were invaluable. Thank you so much.

Jennifer Hubbard: Thank you sincerely for your editing expertise. You always know what I'm trying to say, and you have a special gift in making it come across much more clearly.

Mary Corbett: Your feedback as a fellow nurse practitioner was greatly valued. Thanks also for helping with all the references.

Cynthia Burke Goff: Thank you for keeping the Institute for Integrative Medicine running smoothly when I remained at home writing.

Tara Remington: Thank you for your beautiful illustrations. You captured exactly the essence and spirit of each chapter. You are quite gifted.

Pamela McDonald and Mary Ann Osborne: Words cannot express what the two of you mean to me. I greatly admire both of you as nurse practitioners, entrepreneurs, and certainly movers and shakers in the world of integrative medicine, holistic nursing, wellness, and disease prevention. I am so grateful the universe brought the three of us together to do this work. You are my sisters in healing.

Lucia Thornton: Thank you so much for letting me use your table comparing models of health care practices. I love your *Whole Person Caring* book. We are truly kindred spirits.

Lara Salyer Smith, MD: Thank you for your blog post: "Dear Hippocrates: I Want a Divorce." It's brilliant and such an adequate description of the issues today's healthcare providers must face.

Tracy, Bubba's mother, Debbie, Patrice, Mary Jo, Jeff, Joy, Karen, and Stacy: Thank you all for allowing me to share your stories. Thanks to each of you for your commitment to achieving your optimal health of mind, body, and spirit.

John W. Travis, MD: Thank you for your brilliant suggestions and expertise in editing and proofing. You were just the person I needed to take this manuscript to the next level. I love your sense of humor. Let's do it again.

Dave Evans: I can never express enough my gratitude and deep love for you. Thank you for your patience, encouragement, and unfailing support in all ways and always! You are my soulmate, my partner and the love of my life.

Bibliography

"Acupuncture: Does It Work? For Which Indications?" *The Medical Letter* 48, no. 1234 (2006): 38–39.

Activate Healthcare. "Our Mission and Values." Activate Healthcare website. https://www.activatehealthcare.com/about-us/our-mission-and-values. Accessed October 23, 2017.

Administration on Aging, Administration for Community Living, and US Department of Health and Human Services. "A Profile of Older Americans: 2012."

Aetna Company. "Aetna Reports Fourth-Quarter and Full-Year 2016 Results." Aetna website. https://news.aetna.com/news-releases/aetna-reports-fourth-quarter-and-full-year-2016-results/. Accessed October 23, 2017.

Agnusdei, Donato, and L. Bufalino. "Efficacy of Ipriflavone in Established Osteoporosis and Long-Term Safety." *Calcified Tissue International* 61 (1997): 523–27.

Ahrens, Tom, Valerie Yancey, and Marin Kollef. "Improving Family Communications at the End of Life: Implications for Length of Stay in the Intensive Care Unit and Resource Use." *American Journal of Critical Care* 12, no. 4 (July 2003).

Alexander, Eben. *Proof of Heaven: A Neurosurgeon's Journey into the Afterlife.* New York: Simon & Schuster, 2012.

American Psychological Association. "Stress in America: The State of Our Nation." November 1, 2017. APA website. http://www.apa.org/news/press/releases/stress/2017/state-nation.pdf.

Ammendolia, Carlo, Andrea D. Furlan, Marta Imamura, Emma Irvin, and Maurits van Tulder. "Evidence-Informed Management of Chronic Low Back Pain with Needle Acupuncture." *Spine Journal* 8, no. 1 (2008): 160–72.

Anandarajah, Gowri, and Ellen Hight. "Spirituality and Medical Practice: Using the HOPE Questions as a Practical Tool for Spiritual Assessment." *American Family Physician* 63, no. 1 (2001): 81–89.

Angell, Marcia. *The Truth About Drug Companies: How They Deceive Us and What to Do About It.* New York: Random House, 2005.

"Anthem Revenue, Profits: ANTM Annual Income Statement." Amigo Bulls website. https://amigobulls.com/stocks/ANTM/income-statement/annual. Accessed October 23, 2017.

Arora, Nimmi, Diana Martins, Danielle Ruggerio, Eleni Tousimis, Alexander J. Swistel, Michael P. Osborne, and Rache M. Simmons. "Effectiveness of a Noninvasive Digital Infrared Thermal Imaging System in the Detection of Breast Cancer." *American Journal of Surgery* 196, no. 4 (October 2008): 523–26.

Bakalar, Nicholas. "Prescription Drug Use Soared in Past Decade." *The New York Times*, October 18, 2010. https://www.nytimes.com/2010/10/19/health/research/19stats.html.

Bartol, Genevieve M., and Nancy F. Courts. "The Psychophysiology of Body-Mind Healing." In *Holistic Nursing: A Handbook for Practice.* 6th ed., edited by Barbara Montgomery Dossey and Lynn Keegan. Burlington, NH: Jones & Bartlett, 2013.

Berner, Nathan, and Don Capoferri. "Complete Cervical Kyphosis Correction and Resolution of Low Back Pain Utilizing Pierce Technique." *Annals of Vertebral Subluxation Research* (November 2011): 183–88.

Bernhoft, Robin, and Rashid Buttar. "Autism: A Multi-System Oxidative and Inflammatory Disorder." *Townsend Letter* (April 2008).

Birnbaum, Sam. "Pulmonary Rehabilitation: A Classic Tune with a New Beat, but Is Anyone Listening?" *Chest Journal* 139, no. 6 (2011): 1698.

Block, Keith. Block Center for Integrative Cancer Treatment. http://blockmd.com/. Accessed October 23, 2017.

Bly, Robert. *A Little Book on the Human Shadow.* San Francisco: HarperOne, 1988.

Bowler, Ginger. *Listening and Communicating with Energy.* Madison, WI: Focus on the Light Publishing, 2000.

Bowman, David. "What the Research Says about Thermography: An Annotated Bibliography of Research on Using Thermography for Detecting Breast Cancer." Thermal Imaging of the Southwest website. http://tiofsw.com/wp-content/uploads/2014/08/Scientific-Bibliography-Mammograms.pdf. Accessed October 23, 2017.

Braden, Gregg. *The Divine Matrix: Bridging Time, Space, Miracles, and Belief.* Carlsbad, CA: Hay House, 2007.

Bronfort, Gert, Mitch Haas, Roni Evans, Greg Kawchuk, and Simon Dagenais. "Evidence-Informed Management of Chronic Low Back Pain with Spinal Manipulation and Mobilization." *Spine Journal* 8, no. 1 (2008): 213–25.

Brumleve, Gertrude. "Emotional Maturity: What Is It?" Presentation at Institute for Integrative Medicine, Louisville, KY, September 27, 2002.

Burcon, Michael, and Jennifer Pero. "Resolution of Glossopharyngeal Neuralgia and Spastic Dystonia Following Chiropractic Care to Reduce Upper Cervical Vertebral Subluxation: A Case Study." *Journal of Upper Cervical Chiropractic Research* (January 2014): 7–13.

Burkhardt, Margaret A., and Mary Gail Nagai-Jacobson. "Spirituality and Health." In *Holistic Nursing: A Handbook for Practice.* 6th ed., edited by Barbara Montgomery Dossey and Lynn Keegan. Burlington, NH: Jones & Bartlett, 2013.

Burpo, Todd, with Lynn Vincent. *Heaven Is for Real.* Nashville, TN: HIFR Ministries, 2011.

Campbell, Susan, and John Grey. *Five-Minute Relationship Repair: Quickly Heal Upsets, Deepen Intimacy, and Use Differences to Strengthen Love.* Novato, CA: New World Library, 2015.

Center for Integrative Medicine. University of Arizona. "What is Integrative Medicine?" Center for Integrative Medicine website. https://integrative-medicine.arizona.edu/about/definition.html. Accessed October 23, 2017.

Centers for Disease Control and Prevention. "Chronic Disease Overview." CDC website. https://www.cdc.gov/chronicdisease/overview/index.htm. Accessed October 23, 2017.

———. "Key Elements of Healthy Eating Patterns" in *Dietary Guidelines, 2015–2020.* CDC website. https://health.gov/dietaryguidelines/2015/

guidelines/chapter-1/a-closer-look-inside-healthy-eating-patterns/#callout-dietary-fats. Accessed October 23, 2017.

———. "Leading Causes of Death and Numbers of Deaths, by Sex, Race, and Hispanic Origin: United States, 1980 and 2014 (Table 19)." In *Health, United States, 2015*. CDC website https://www.cdc.gov/nchs/data/hus/hus15.pdf#019. Accessed October 23, 2017.

———. National Center for Health Statistics, "Therapeutic Drug Use," CDC website, https://www.cdc.gov/nchs/fastats/drug-use-therapeutic.htm, accessed October 23, 2017.

———. "Preventable Deaths from Heart Disease and Stroke." CDC website. https://www.cdc.gov/vitalsigns/HeartDisease-Stroke/index.html. Accessed October 23, 2017.

———. "Vaccine Safety. Thimerosal in Vaccines." CDC website: https://www.cdc.gov/vaccinesafety/concerns/thimerosal/. Accessed October 23, 2017.

Centers for Medicare and Medicaid Services. "National Health Expenditure Data." Centers for Medicare and Medicaid Services website. www.cms.gov/Research-Statistics-Data-and-Systems/Statistics-Trends-and-Reports/NationalHealthExpendData/NationalHealthAccountsHistorical.html.

Chapman, Cheryl. *The Happy Breast Book: A Women's Guide to Keeping Your Breasts Healthy and Happy*. Maplewood, NJ: Cheryl Chapman, 2003.

"Cigna Revenue, Profits: CI Annual Income Statement." Amigo Bulls website. https://amigobulls.com/stocks/CI/income-statement/annual. Accessed October 23, 2017.

Committee on the Robert Wood Johnson Foundation Initiative on the Future of Nursing. *The Future of Nursing: Leading Change, Advancing Health*. Washington, DC: Institute of Medicine/National Academies Press, 2011. https://www.nap.edu/read/12956/chapter/1. Accessed October 23, 2017.

"Corn, Corn, Everywhere Corn." Institute for Responsible Technology website. https://responsibletechnology.org/corn-corn-everywhere-corn/. Accessed October 23, 2017.

"Corn Products and Derivatives List." Institute for Responsible Technology website. https://responsibletechnology.org/irtnew/wp-content/uploads/2017/06/Corn-Products-Derivatives-06-06-17.pdf. Accessed October 23, 2017.

Cotman, Carl. "Diet and Exercise in Alzheimer's." Part of *The Alzheimer's Project,* a presentation of HBO Documentary Films and the National Institute on Aging at the National Institutes of Health. 2009.

Davis, Karen, Kristof Stremikis, D. Squires, and Cathy Schoen. "Mirror, Mirror on the Wall: How the Performance of the US Health Care System Compares Internationally." *The Commonwealth Fund.* 2014.

de Botton, Alain. "Why You Will Marry the Wrong Person." *New York Times* website. https://www.nytimes.com/2016/05/29/opinion/sunday/why-you-will-marry-the-wrong-person.html. Accessed October 23, 2017.

Donaldson, Michael S. "Nutrition and Cancer: A Review of the Evidence for an Anti-Cancer Diet." *Nutrition Journal* 19 (October 2004).

Dossey, Barbara Montgomery, and Lynn Keegan. "Nursing: Integral, Integrative, and Holistic: Local to Global." In *Holistic Nursing: A Handbook for Practice.* 6th ed., edited by Barbara Montgomery Dossey and Lynn Keegan. Burlington, NH: Jones & Bartlett, 2013.

Dossey, Larry. *Healing Words: The Power of Prayer and the Practice of Medicine.* New York: Harper Collins, 1993.

Dyer, Wayne W. *There's a Spiritual Solution to Every Problem.* Carlsbad, CA: Hay House, 2002.

———. *The Power of Intention: Learning to Co-Create Your World Your Way.* Carlsbad, CA: Hay House, 2010.

Eenfeldt, Andreas. "The Hidden Truth Behind Ancel Keys' Famous Fat Graph." September 19, 2016. Diet Doctor website. https://www.dietdoctor.com/the-hidden-truth-behind-ancel-keys-famous-fat-graph.

Ehrmann, Max. "Desiderata." All Poetry website. https://allpoetry.com/Desiderata---Words-for-Life. Originally published 1927. Accessed October 23, 2017.

Environmental Protection Agency, Office of Pesticide Programs. "Glyphosate Issue Paper: Evaluation of Carcinogenic Potential." September 12, 2016. EPA website. https://www.epa.gov/sites/production/files/2016-09/documents/glyphosate_issue_paper_evaluation_of_carcincogenic_potential.pdf.

Epstein, Samuel S. "Hormones in US Beef Linked to Increased Cancer Risk." October 21, 2009. Organic Consumers Association website. https://www.organicconsumers.org/news/hormones-us-beef-linked-increased-cancer-risk.

Estes, Tarron, Conscious Dying Institute website. http://www. consciousdyinginstitute.com/. Accessed October 23, 2017.

Evans, Kimberly A. (Genevieve Bartol and Nancy F. Courts, original authors.) "The Psychophysiology of Body-Mind Healing." In *Core Curriculum for Holistic Nursing*, 2nd ed., edited by Mary Helming, Cynthia C. Barrere, Karen Avino, and Deborah Shields. Burlington, MA: Jones & Bartlett, 2014.

Flavin, Dana. "Metabolic Dangers of High-Fructose Corn Syrup." *Life Extension* magazine website. http://www.lifeextension.com/ magazine/2008/12/Metabolic-Dangers-of-High-Fructose-Corn-Syrup/ Page-01. Accessed October 23, 2017.

Food, Inc. Robin Schorr, Jeff Skoll, and Diane Weyermann, executive producers; Robert Kenner, director and producer. Magnolia Pictures, 2008. Documentary film.

Forks over Knives. Brian Wendel, executive producer; Lee Fulkerson, director. Monica Beach Media, 2011. Documentary film.

Fox, Nick J., and Katie J. Ward. "Pharma in the Bedroom . . . and the Kitchen . . . The Pharmaceuticalisation of Daily Life." *Sociology of Health & Illness* 30, no. 6 (September 2008): 856–68.

Gasnier, Céline, Coralie Dumont, Nora Benachour, Emilie Clair, Marie-Christine Chagnon, and Gilles-Eric Séralini. "Glyphosate-Based Herbicides Are Toxic and Endocrine Disruptors in Human Cell Lines." *Toxicology* 262, no. 3 (August 21, 2009): 184–91.

Gawande Atul. "The Checklist." *New Yorker Magazine: Annals of Medicine*, December 10, 2007. https://newyorker.com/magazine/2007/12/10/the-checklist.

———. "Can Life in a Nursing Home Be Uplifting?" October 4, 2014. *The Telegraph* website. https://www.telegraph.co.uk/culture/books/11139446/ Can-life-in-a-nursing-home-be-made-uplifting-and-purposeful.html.

———. *Being Mortal: Medicine and What Matters in the End.* New York: Picador, 2017.

———. *The Checklist Manifesto: How to Get Things Right.* New York: Picador, 2011.

Geier, David A., Paul G. King, and Mark R. Geier. "Mitochondrial Dysfunction, Impaired Oxidative-Reduction Activity, Degeneration, and Death in Human Neuronal and Fetal Cells Induced by Low-Level

Exposure to Thimerosal and Other Metal Compounds." *Toxicological and Environmental Chemistry* 91, no. 3–4 (2009): 735–49.

Gerards, Maaike C., Ruben J. Terlou, Huixin Yu, C. H. W. Koks, and V. E. A. Gerdes. "Traditional Chinese Lipid-Lowering Agent Red Yeast Rice Results in Significant LDL Reduction but Safety Is Uncertain: A Systematic Review and Meta-Analysis." *Atherosclerosis* 240, no. 2 (June 2015): 415–23.

Godfrey, M. E., D. P. Wojcik, and C. A. Krone. "Apolipoprotein E Genotyping as a Potential Biomarker for Mercury Neurotoxicity." *Journal of Alzheimer's Disease* 5, no. 3 (June 2003): 189–95. http://www. optimalfunctioning.com/research/godfrey-et-al-2003-apolipoprotein-e-genotyping-as-potential-biomarker-for-mercury-neurotoxicity.html.

Goetz Christine M., Cynthia R. Long, Maria A. Hondras, Richard Petri, Roxana Delgado, Dana J. Lawrence, Edward Owens, and William C. Meeker. "Adding Chiropractic Manipulative Therapy to Standard Medical Care for Patients with Acute Low Back Pain: Results of a Pragmatic Randomized Comparative Effectiveness Study." *Spine* 38, no. 8 (April 2013): 627–34.

Goldhill, David. "How American Healthcare Killed My Father." *The Atlantic*. September 2009. https://www.theatlantic.com/magazine/archive/2009/09/how-american-health-care-killed-my-father/307617/. Accessed October 23, 2017.

———. *Catastrophic Care: Why Everything We Think We Know about Healthcare Is Wrong*. New York: First Vintage Books, 2013.

Gu, Qiuping, Charles F. Dillon, and Vicki L. Burt. "Prescription Drug Use Continues to Increase: US Prescription Drug Data for 2007–2008." *NCHS Data Brief* 42 (September 2010): 1–8.

Haley, Boyd E., and Teri Small. "Interview with Dr. Boyd E. Haley: Biomarkers Supporting Mercury Toxicity as the Major Exacerbator of Neurological Illness, Recent Evidence via the Urinary Porphyrin Tests." *Medical Veritas* 3 (2006): 921–34.

HeartMath® Institute. "Solutions for Stress." HeartMath® Institute website. https://www.HeartMath®.org/resources/solutions-for-stress/reducing-stress/. Accessed October 23, 2017.

———. "Top Tips for Better Sleep." HeartMath® Institute website. https://www.HeartMath®.com/articles/top-tips-for-better-sleep/. Accessed October 23, 2017.

Hearts in Healthcare. https://heartsinhealthcare.com/. Accessed October 23, 2017.

Heyes, G. J., A. J. Mill, and Monty W. Charles. "Enhanced Biological Effectiveness of Low Energy X-rays and Implications for the UK Breast Screening Programme." *British Journal of Radiology* 79, no. 939 (March 2006): 195–200.

"Humana Revenue, Profits: HUM Annual Income Statement." Amigo Bulls website. https://amigobulls.com/stocks/HUM/income-statement/annual. Accessed October 23, 2017.

Imamura, Marta, Andrea D. Furlan, Trish Dryden, and Emma Irvin. "Evidence-Informed Management of Chronic Low Back Pain with Massage." *Spine Journal* 8, no. 1 (2008): 121–33.

Institute of Medicine. "Dietary Reference Intakes: Electrolytes and Water." National Agricultural Library, United States Department of Agriculture website. https://www.nal.usda.gov/sites/default/files/fnic_uploads//electrolytes_water.pdf. Accessed October 23, 2017.

Kaiser Family Foundation website. https://www.kff.org/.

Katon, Wayne, and Ed Walker. "Medically Unexplained Symptoms in Primary Care." *Journal of Clinical Psychology* 59, supplement 20 (1998): 15–21.

Kennedy, Patrick. "CEO Pay Watch: UnitedHealth's Stephen Hemsley Made $31.3 Million Last Year." April 24, 2017. http://www.startribune.com/CEO-pay-watch-unitedhealth-s-stephen-hemsley-made-31-3-million-last-year/420284643/.

Klimek, Matthew, Shan Wang, and Adeleye Ogunkanmi. "Safety and Efficacy of Red Yeast Rice *(Monascus purpureus)* as an Alternative Therapy for Hyperlipemia." *Pharmacy & Therapuetics* 34, no. 6 (2009): 313–27.

Knapen, Marjo H. J., Nadja E. A. Drummen, E. Smit, C. Vermeer, and Elke Theuwissen. "Three-Year Low-Dose Menaquinone-7 Supplementation Helps Decrease Bone Loss in Healthy Postmenopausal Women." *Osteoporosis International* 24, no. 9 (September 2013): 2499–507.

Kohn, Linda T., Janet M. Corrigan, and Molla S. Donaldson. "To Err Is Human: Building a Safer Health System." Washington, DC: Institute of Medicine/National Academies Press, 2000.

Kübler Ross, Elisabeth, and Ira Byock. *On Death and Dying: What the Dying Have to Teach Doctors, Nurses, Clergy and Their Own Families.* New York: Scribner, 2011.

Kuhn, Clifford. *It All Starts with a Smile*. Louisville, KY: Butler Books, 2007.

Kushner, Robert F., Linda Van Horn, Cheryl L. Rock, Marilyn S. Edwards, Connie W. Bales, Martin Kohlmeier, and Sharon R. Akabas. "Nutrition Education in Medical School: A Time of Opportunity." *American Journal of Clinical Nutrition* 99, no. 5 (2014): 1167S–73S.

Leo, Pam. *Connection Parenting: Parenting through Connection Instead of Coercion, through Love Instead of Fear*. 2nd ed. Deadwood, OR: Wyatt-MacKenzie, 2007.

Lipton, Bruce. *The Biology of Belief: Unleashing the Power of Consciousness, Matter, and Miracles*. Carlsbad, CA: Hay House, 2007.

Makary, Martin A., and Michael Daniel. "Medical Error: The Third Leading Cause of Death in the US." *BMJ* (May 2016) 353:i2139.

Maugeri, Domenico, Pietra Panebianco, Mario S. Russo, Massimo Motta, Salvatore Tropea, L. Cayolla da Motta, C. Garozzo, et. al. "Ipriflavone Treatment of Senile Osteoporosis: Results of a Multicenter, Double-Blind Clinical Trial of Two Years." *Archives of Gerontology and Geriatrics* 19, no. 3 (November–December 1994): 253–63.

Mayer, John M., Vert Mooney, and Simon Dagenais. "Evidence-Informed Management of Chronic Low Back Pain with Chronic Lumbar Extensor Strengthening Exercises." *Spine Journal* 8, no. 1 (2008): 96–113.

Mayo Clinic. "Dementia." Mayo Clinic website. https://www.mayoclinic.org/diseases-conditions/dementia/symptoms-causes/syc-20352013. Accessed October 23, 2017.

McCullough, Marjorie. "Preventing Cancer with Food: Magic Bullets vs. Dietary Patterns." Presented at the 7th Annual Nutrition and Health Conference, May 11, 2010. Atlanta, GA. file:///C:/Users/Susan/AppData/Local/Temp/NHC2010-online_brochure.pdf. Accessed October 23, 2017.

McDonald, Pamela. APO E Gene website. https://apoegenediet.com/. Accessed October 23, 2017.

———. *The Perfect Gene Diet*. Carlsbad, CA: Hay House, 2010.

McLeod, Saul. "Maslow's Hierarchy of Needs." https://simplypsychology.org/maslow.html. Accessed October 23, 2017.

Mentes, Janet. "Oral Hydration in Older Adults: Greater Awareness is Needed in Preventing, Recognizing, and Treating Dehydration." *American Journal of Nursing* 106, no. 6 (2006): 40–49.

Mercola, Joseph. *Fat for Fuel: A Revolutionary Diet to Combat Cancer, Boost Brain Power, and Increase Your Energy*. Carlsbad, CA: Hay House, 2017.

Miller, Elaine Tilka, Carol Deets, and Robert V. Miller. "Nurse Call Systems: Impact on Nursing Performance." *Journal of Nursing Care Quality* 11, no. 3 (1997): 36-43.

"Mission, Vision, Values, Principles." Eden Alternative website. http://www.edenalt.org/about-the-eden-alternative/mission-vision-values/. Accessed October 23, 2017.

Moorjani, Anita. *Dying to Be Me: My Journey from Cancer, to Near Death, to True Healing*. Carlsbad, CA: Hay House, 2012.

Motz, J. "Everyone an Energy Healer: The Treat V Conference Santa Fe, NM," *The Journal of Mind-Body Health* 9 (1993).

Murphy, Jonathan, Timothy Morrison, Rod Floyd, and Joel Alcantara. "Improvement in a Patient with Disc Protrusion and Extruded Fragment Following Subluxation-Based Chiropractic Care: A Case Study and Selective Review of the Literature." *Annals of Vertebral Subluxation Research* (November 2015): 178–83.

Nance, John J., and Kathleen M. Bartholomew. *Charting the Course: Launching Patient-Centric Healthcare*. Bozeman, MT: Second River Healthcare Press, 2012.

National Center for Complementary and Integrative Health. "NCCIH Facts at a Glance and Mission." NCCIH website. https://nccih.nih.gov/about/ataglance. Accessed October 23, 2017.

———. "Research Results." NCCIH website. https://nccih.nih.gov/research/results. Accessed October 23, 2017.

———. "Herbs at a Glance." NCCIH website. https://nccih.nih.gov/health/herbsataglance.htm. Accessed October 23, 2017.

National Coalition on Health Care website. https://nchc.org/.

Ng, Eddie Y. K. "A Review of Thermography as Promising Non-Invasive Detection Modality for Breast Tumor." *International Journal of Thermal Sciences* 48 (May 2009): 849–59.

Non-GMO Shopping Guide website. https://www.nongmoshoppingguide.com/. Accessed October 23, 2017.

Ornish, Dean. *Dr. Dean Ornish's Program for Reversing Heart Disease: The Only System Scientifically Proven to Reverse Heart Disease without Drugs or Surgery.* New York: Random House, 1990.

Perkins, A. "Saving Money by Reducing Stress." *Harvard Business Review* 72, no. 6 (1994): 12.

Pijpe, Anouk, Nadine Andrieu, Douglas F. Easton, Ausrele Kesminiene, Elisabeth Cardis, Catherine Noguès, Marion Gauthier-Villars, et al. "Exposure to Diagnostic Radiation and Risk of Breast Cancer among Carriers of BRCA1/2 Mutations: Retrospective Cohort Study (GENE-RAD-RISK)." *BMJ* 345 (2012): e5660.

Piper, Don, with Cecil Murphey. *90 Minutes in Heaven: A True Story of Death and Life.* Grand Rapids, MI: Revell, 2004.

Planetree Alliance website. https://planetree.org/. Accessed October 23, 2017.

"Proclamation for Transforming the Lives of Children." Alliance for Transforming the Lives of Children website. http://atlc.org/Proclamation/proclamation.php. Accessed October 23, 2017.

Pronovost, Peter, Dale Needham, Sean Berenholtz, David Sinopoli, Haitao Chu, Sara Cosgrove, Bryan Sexton, et al. "An Intervention to Decrease Catheter-Related Bloodstream Infections in the ICU." *New England Journal of Medicine* 355 (2006): 2725–32.

Rassiwala, Muffazzal, Poonam Mathur, Rajkumar K. Mathur, K. S. Farid, Sapna Shukla, Prabodh K. Gupta, and Beena Jain. "Evaluation of Digital Infra-Red Thermal Imaging as an Adjunctive Screening Method for Breast Carcinoma: A Pilot Study." *International Journal of Surgery* 12 (December 2014): 1439–43.

Rivera, A. Joy, and Ben-Tzion Karsh. "Interruptions and Distractions in Healthcare: Review and Reappraisal." *Quality and Safety in Health Care* 19, no. 4 (2010): 304–12.

Roizman, Tracey. "Do Hormones in the Food Supply Affect the Human Body?" *SF GATE.* https://healthyeating.sfgate.com/hormones-food-supply-affect-human-body-2194.html. Accessed October 23, 2017.

Rosenboro, Ken. "Why Is Glyphosate Sprayed on Crops Right Before Harvest?" Eco Watch website, March 6, 2016. https://www.ecowatch.com/why-is-glyphosate-sprayed-on-crops-right-before-harvest-1882187755.html. Accessed October 23, 2017.

Rozman, Deborah, and Rollin McCraty. *HeartMath® Solution for Better Sleep: Resetting Your Body's Rhythms, Integrating emWave and Inner Balance Technologies.* Boulder Creek, CA: HeartMath® LLC, 2013.

Salyer, Lara. "Dear Hippocrates: I Want a Divorce." August 13, 2016. Kevin MD website. https://www.kevinmd.com/blog/2016/08/dear-hippocrates-want-divorce.html.

Samsel, Anthony, and Stephanie Seneff. "Glyphosate's Suppression of Cytochrome P450 Enzymes and Amino Acid Biosynthesis by the Gut Microbiome: Pathways to Modern Diseases." *Entropy* 15, no. 4 (2013): 1416–63.

Saputo, Len. *A Return to Healing: Radical Healthcare Reform and the Future of Medicine.* San Rafael, CA: Origin Press, 2009.

Schaafsma, Anne, P. J. F. de Vries, and W. H. M. Saris. "Delay of Natural Bone Loss by Higher Intakes of Specific Minerals and Vitamins." *Critical Reviews in Food Science and Nutrition* 41, no. 4 (May 2001): 225–49.

Self-Nutrition Data. "Glycemic Index." Self-Nutrition Data website. http://nutritiondata.self.com/topics/glycemic-index. Accessed October 23, 2017.

Shaw, Christopher A., Stephanie Seneff, Stephen D. Kette, Lucija Tomljenovic, John W. Oller Jr., and Robert M. Davidson. "Aluminum-Induced Entropy in Biological Systems: Implications for Neurological Disease." *Journal of Toxicology* (2014) http://dx.doi.org/10.1155/2014/491316.

"Shopper's Guide to Pesticides in Produce: Clean Fifteen and Dirty Dozen Foods." Environmental Working Group website. https://www.ewg.org/foodnews/. Accessed October 23, 2017.

Small, Leslie. "Health Insurance CEO Pay Tops Out at $17.3M in 2015." April 24, 2016. Fierce Healthcare website. https://www.fiercehealthcare.com/payer/health-insurance-CEO-pay-at-big-five-tops-out-at-17-3m-2015.

Smith, Jeffrey M. "Are Genetically Modified Foods a Gut-Wrenching Combination?" Institute for Responsible Technology website. http://responsibletechnology.org/glutenintroduction/. Accessed October 23, 2017.

———. "GMO FAQs." Institute for Responsible Technology website. http://responsibletechnology.org/gmo-education/faqs/. Accessed October 23, 2017.

———. *Seeds of Deception. Exposing Industry and Government Lies About the Safety of the Genetically Engineered Foods You're Eating.* Fairfield, IA: Yes! Books, 2002.

Sree, Vinitah, E. Y. K. Ng, Rajendra U. Acharya, and O. Faust. "Breast Imaging: A Survey." *World Journal of Clinical Oncology* 2, no. 4 (2011): 171–78.

Stone, Gene, ed. *Forks over Knives: The Plant-Based Way to Health.* New York: The Experiment, 2011.

Taylor, Ginger. "142 Research Papers Supporting Vaccine/ Autism Causation." SCRIBD website, https://www.scribd.com/ doc/220807175/150-Research-Papers-Supporting-the-Vaccine-Autism-Link. Accessed October 23, 2017.

Thornton, Lucia. *Whole Person Caring: An Interprofessional Model for Healing and Wellness.* Indianapolis: Sigma Theta Tau International, 2013.

Tomljenovic Lucija, and C. Shaw. "Aluminum Vaccine Adjuvants: Are They Safe?" *Current Medicinal Chemistry* 18 (2011): 2630–37.

Tucker, Anita L. "The Impact of Operational Failures on Hospital Nurses and Their Patients." *Journal of Operations Management* 22, no. 2 (2004): 151–69.

Tucker, Anita L., and Steven J. Spear. "Operational Failures and Interruptions in Hospital Nursing." *Health Services Research* 42 (2006): 643–62.

United Health Group. "Unitedhealth Group Reports 2016 Results Highlighted by Continued Strong and Diversified Growth." United Health Group website. https://unitedhealthgroup.com/content/dam/ UHG/PDF/investors/2016/UNH-Q4-2016-Release.pdf. Accessed October 23, 2017.

United States Census Bureau. "Statistical Abstract of the US: 1989." US Census Bureau website. https://www.census.gov/library/ publications/1989/compendia/statab/109ed.html.

Vital Choice website. https://www.vitalchoice.com/. Accessed October 23, 2017.

Walker, Brad. "The FITT Principle: Frequency, Intensity, Time, Type and How They Relate to Injury." Stretch Coach website. http://stretchcoach. com/articles/fitt-principle/. First published September 24, 2003; updated May 23, 2017; accessed October 23, 2017.

Ward, Brian W., Jeannine S. Schiller, and Richard A. Goodman. "Multiple Chronic Conditions Among US Adults: A 2012 Update." *Preventing Chronic Disease* 11 (2014): 130389.

Weil, Andrew. "Dr. Weil's Anti-Inflammatory Food Pyramid." Dr. Weil's website. https://www.drweil.com/diet-nutrition/anti-inflammatory-diet-pyramid/dr-weils-anti-inflammatory-food-pyramid/. Accessed October 23, 2017.

———. "Three Breathing Exercises and Techniques." Dr. Weil's website. https://www.drweil.com/health-wellness/body-mind-spirit/stress-anxiety/breathing-three-exercises/. Accessed October 23, 2017.

———. *Why Our Health Matters: A Vision of Medicine That Can Transform Our Future.* New York: Hudson Street Press, 2009.

Wikipedia. "Chinese Word for Crisis." https://en.wikipedia.org/wiki/Chinese_word_for_%22crisis%22. Accessed October 23, 2017.

"Workplace Stress." American Institute of Stress website. https://www.stress.org/workplace-stress/. Accessed October 23, 2017.

World Health Organization. Constitution as Adopted by the International Health Conference, New York, June 19–22, 1946. WHO website. http://www.who.int/about/mission/en/. Accessed October 23, 2017.

———. *The World Health Report 2000—Health Systems: Improving Performance.* Geneva, Switzerland: World Health Organization, 2000.

Youngson, Robin. *Time to Care: How to Love Your Patients and Your Job.* New Zealand: Rebelheart Publishers, 2012.

Zhang, Xin, Shao-wen Li, Jin-Fang Wu, Chun-Li Dong, Cai-xia Zheng, Yun-ping Zhang, and Juan Du. "Effects of Ipriflavone on Postmenopausal Syndrome and Osteoporosis." *Gynecological Endocrinology* 26, no. 2 (2010).

About the Author

Kim Evans is an advanced practice clinical nurse specialist (APRN), certified in adult health nursing. She has an extensive clinical background including staff nurse, nurse manager, critical care clinical nurse specialist, and nurse entrepreneur. She has worked in various clinical areas including transitional care, emergency room, respiratory intensive care, coronary care, open heart surgery, and as a critical care nurse specialist.

After an epiphany in the intensive care unit one day, she realized that 80 percent of the patients in the ICU had illnesses that could have been prevented. From that day forward, she focused her practice on disease prevention, wellness, and achieving optimal health of mind, body, and spirit. She is certified in advanced holistic nursing practice (American Holistic Nurses Credentialing Corporation) and Amma Therapy (New York College of Holistic Health, Education, and Research) and has completed the Fellowship in Integrative Medicine through the University of Arizona with Andrew Weil, MD.

Kim is a founding member of the Institute for Integrative Medicine in Louisville, Kentucky, which has grown from its humble beginnings to include 10 practitioners, all experts in their fields. She has authored multiple articles and book chapters on clinical nursing, holistic nursing, integrative medicine, and wellness.

She is married to the love of her life, Dave, and together they have six children, two daughters-in-law, and five grandchildren. They each come from large extended families, which they love dearly. In her free time, she enjoys hiking, boating, playing tennis, and traveling to Hawaii to visit her children. She has a passion for college football and basketball, especially the Louisville Cardinals.

Kim is available for consultation, workshops, seminars, retreats, and keynote speaking engagements. Check out her website at www. integrativemedicine4u.com or contact her at her office:

Institute for Integrative Medicine
205 Townepark Circle, Suite 100
Louisville, KY 40243
(502) 253-4554